COVID-19: Impact on Public Health and Healthcare (Volume 2)

COVID-19: Impact on Public Health and Healthcare (Volume 2)

Editors

Kavita Batra
Manoj Sharma

MDPI • Basel • Beijing • Wuhan • Barcelona • Belgrade • Manchester • Tokyo • Cluj • Tianjin

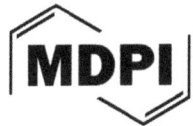

Editors
Kavita Batra
Kirk Kerkorian School of Medicine at University of Nevada
USA

Manoj Sharma
University of Nevada
USA

Editorial Office
MDPI
St. Alban-Anlage 66
4052 Basel, Switzerland

This is a reprint of articles from the Topical Collection published online in the open access journal *Healthcare* (ISSN 2227-9032) (available at: https://www.mdpi.com/journal/healthcare/special_issues/covid-19_publichealth).

For citation purposes, cite each article independently as indicated on the article page online and as indicated below:

LastName, A.A.; LastName, B.B.; LastName, C.C. Article Title. *Journal Name* **Year**, *Volume Number*, Page Range.

ISBN 978-3-0365-2844-1 (Hbk)
ISBN 978-3-0365-2845-8 (PDF)

© 2021 by the authors. Articles in this book are Open Access and distributed under the Creative Commons Attribution (CC BY) license, which allows users to download, copy and build upon published articles, as long as the author and publisher are properly credited, which ensures maximum dissemination and a wider impact of our publications.

The book as a whole is distributed by MDPI under the terms and conditions of the Creative Commons license CC BY-NC-ND.

Contents

About the Editors vii

Preface to "COVID-19: Impact on Public Health and Healthcare (Volume 2)" ix

Kavita Batra, Manoj Sharma, Ravi Batra, Tejinder Pal Singh and Nena Schvaneveldt
Assessing the Psychological Impact of COVID-19 among College Students: An Evidence of 15 Countries
Reprinted from: *Healthcare* **2021**, *9*, 222, doi:10.3390/healthcare9020222 1

Yin Li, Linbo Qin, Yaobin Shi and Jun Han
The Psychological Symptoms of College Student in China during the Lockdown of COVID-19 Epidemic
Reprinted from: *Healthcare* **2021**, *9*, 447, doi:10.3390/healthcare9040447 19

Jaewon Lee, Jennifer Allen, Hyejung Lim and Gyuhyun Choi
Determinants of Behavioral Changes Since COVID-19 among Middle School Students
Reprinted from: *Healthcare* **2021**, *9*, 75, doi:10.3390/healthcare9010075 29

Abdullah Alassaf, Basim Almulhim, Sara Ayid Alghamdi and Sreekanth Kumar Mallineni
Perceptions and Preventive Practices Regarding COVID-19 Pandemic Outbreak and Oral Health Care Perceptions during the Lockdown: A Cross-Sectional Survey from Saudi Arabia
Reprinted from: *Healthcare* **2021**, *9*, 959, doi:10.3390/healthcare9080959 39

Ji Liu, Baihuiyu Li, Qiaoyi Chen and Jingxia Dang
Student Health Implications of School Closures during the COVID-19 Pandemic: New Evidence on the Association of e-Learning, Outdoor Exercise, and Myopia
Reprinted from: *Healthcare* **2021**, *9*, 500, doi:10.3390/healthcare9050500 53

André Hajek, Freia De Bock, Lena Huebl, Benedikt Kretzler and Hans-Helmut König
Postponed Dental Visits during the COVID-19 Pandemic and their Correlates. Evidence from the Nationally Representative COVID-19 Snapshot Monitoring in Germany (COSMO)
Reprinted from: *Healthcare* **2021**, *9*, 50, doi:10.3390/healthcare9010050 63

Reidar P. Lystad, Benjamin T. Brown, Michael S. Swain and Roger M. Engel
Impact of the COVID-19 Pandemic on Manual Therapy Service Utilization within the Australian Private Healthcare Setting
Reprinted from: *Healthcare* **2020**, *8*, 558, doi:10.3390/healthcare8040558 73

Syed Mohammed Basheeruddin Asdaq, Sara Abdulrahman Alajlan, Yahya Mohzari, Mohammed Asad, Ahmad Alamer, Ahmed A. Alrashed, Naira Nayeem and Sreeharsha Nagaraja
COVID-19 and Psychological Health of Female Saudi Arabian Population: A Cross-Sectional Study
Reprinted from: *Healthcare* **2020**, *8*, 542, doi:10.3390/healthcare8040542 83

Ramona Bongelli, Carla Canestrari, Alessandra Fermani, Morena Muzi, Ilaria Riccioni, Alessia Bertolazzi and Roberto Burro
Associations between Personality Traits, Intolerance of Uncertainty, Coping Strategies, and Stress in Italian Frontline and Non-Frontline HCWs during the COVID-19 Pandemic—A Multi-Group Path-Analysis
Reprinted from: *Healthcare* **2021**, *9*, 1086, doi:10.3390/healthcare9081086 93

Saad Alyahya and Fouad AboGazalah
Work-Related Stressors among the Healthcare Professionals in the Fever Clinic Centers for Individuals with Symptoms of COVID-19
Reprinted from: *Healthcare* **2021**, *9*, 548, doi:10.3390/healthcare9050548 . . . . **113**

About the Editors

Kavita Batra, PhD, MPH, BDS serves as a Research Biostatistician with the Kirk Kerkorian School of Medicine at the University of Nevada, Las Vegas (UNLV). Dr. Batra received her Ph.D. in Global and Environmental Health from UNLV. Her research interests include maternal and child health, the impact of COVID-19, and disparities among racial and gender minorities. Dr. Batra is an expert in qualitative and quantitative research and has presented her work in several state and national public health conferences. She has published multiple peer-reviewed articles to investigate the impact of COVID-19 on mental health, social connectedness, and employment vulnerability among different demographic and workforce groups. Dr. Batra's recent work related to COVID-19 has been featured in reputed outlets, such as Medscape and Inside Higher Ed. Currently, she is editing three special issues with the *Healthcare* journal. She also serves as a key member to the Nevada Taskforce on Sexual Misconduct.

Manoj Sharma, MBBS, Ph.D., MCHES® is currently a tenured Full Professor and Chair of the Department of Social & Behavioral Health at University of Nevada, Las Vegas, School of Public Health. He is a prolific researcher and has published 11 books, over 325 peer-reviewed research articles, and over 450 other publications and secured funding for over USD 8 million (h-index 44, i-10 index over 175, and over 10,000 citations). He has been awarded several prestigious honors including American Public Health Association's Mentoring Award, ICTHP Impact Award, and J. Mayhew Derryberry Award and William R. Gemma Distinguished Alumnus Award, from the College of Public Health Alumni Society (Ohio State University) among others. His research interests are in developing and evaluating theory-based health behavior change interventions, obesity prevention, stress-coping, community-based participatory research, and integrative mind–body–spirit interventions.

Preface to "COVID-19: Impact on Public Health and Healthcare (Volume 2)"

The coronavirus disease (COVID-19) started in December 2019 and remains a global threat to this day. All dimensions of health, including physical, mental, social, and economic, were severely affected by the COVID-19 pandemic. During the early course of the pandemic, social and physical distancing mandates, including the lockdowns of business, social life, and schools, were critical in limiting the spread. Instituting such non-pharmacologic and public health measures was the only resort, when no or very limited information was available about COVID-19 contagion. The impact of COVID-19 has not been felt uniformly across society; in fact, it has widened pre-existing structural and social inequalities. Youths, older adults, minority groups, persons with disabilities, and essential workers bear a disproportionate burden of the devastating effects of COVID-19. These effects are not short-term; instead, these effects have a far-ranging direct or indirect impact on people lives and well-being. For instance, the disruption in education and sudden transition to online instruction posed significant challenges to students' learning and quality of education. With the economic recession induced by COVID-19, many workers were laid off and faced financial hardships. There were limited job opportunities available in the market. The burden of psychological distress, anxiety, depression, and stress amidst the COVID-19 pandemic was significantly high, which caused young people to adopt negative coping strategies such as substance use, alcohol abuse, underage drinking, and suicidal ideation. During these times, research plays a vital role in shaping each step of the public health response to the pandemic. If the current state is known and understood, preventive strategies can be planned effectively with the aid of collaborative thinking and long-term horizons, with a view to solving one of the world's greatest challenges—the COVID-19 pandemic.

This compendium of studies conducted from around the world focuses on the assessment of the impact of the COVID-19 pandemic. This book begins with a comprehensive meta-analysis of studies from 15 countries assessing the psychological impact of the COVID-19 pandemic among college students. This is followed by a cross-sectional study performed in Wuhan, China to assess the mental status of students during the lockdown period in the COVID-19 pandemic. The behavioral changes among Middle School students are also reported in one of the studies included in this collection. The next study is an assessment of perceptions and preventive practices pertaining to the COVID-19 pandemic and oral health care during the lockdown in Saudi Arabia. This is followed by another China-based study, which assesses the impact of school closures during the COVID-19 pandemic and deciphers association of virtual learning, outdoor exercise, and Myopia. The next two studies measure the impact of COVID-19 on healthcare services, including dental visits and manual therapy utilization in private health care settings. One study from Saudi Arabia summarizes the results of a cross-sectional survey assessing the impact on the mental health of women during the COVID-19 pandemic. Next, a multigroup path analysis approach focuses on coping strategies for frontline as well as non-frontline healthcare workers. Lastly, work-related stressors among healthcare professionals in the fever clinic centers are also included in this book, which also recommends targeted interventions to foster post traumatic growth in this group.

Kavita Batra, Manoj Sharma
Editors

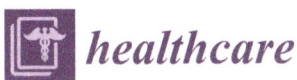

Article

Assessing the Psychological Impact of COVID-19 among College Students: An Evidence of 15 Countries

Kavita Batra [1,*], Manoj Sharma [2], Ravi Batra [3], Tejinder Pal Singh [4] and Nena Schvaneveldt [5]

1. Office of Research, School of Medicine, University of Nevada, Las Vegas, NV 89102, USA
2. Department of Environmental and Occupational Health, University of Nevada, Las Vegas, NV 89119, USA; manoj.sharma@unlv.edu
3. Department of Information Technology and Testing Center of Excellence, Coforge, Atlanta, GA 30338, USA; ravi.batra@coforgetech.com
4. Department of Family and Preventive Medicine, Division of Public Health, School of Medicine, University of Utah, Salt Lake City, UT 84108, USA; tp.singh@utah.edu
5. Spencer S. Eccles Health Sciences Library, University of Utah, Salt Lake City, UT 84112, USA; nena.schvaneveldt@utah.edu
* Correspondence: Kavita.batra@unlv.edu

Citation: Batra, K.; Sharma, M.; Batra, R.; Singh, T.P.; Schvaneveldt, N. Assessing the Psychological Impact of COVID-19 among College Students: An Evidence of 15 Countries. *Healthcare* **2021**, *9*, 222. https://doi.org/10.3390/healthcare9020222

Academic Editor: Alyx Taylor

Received: 27 January 2021
Accepted: 13 February 2021
Published: 17 February 2021

Publisher's Note: MDPI stays neutral with regard to jurisdictional claims in published maps and institutional affiliations.

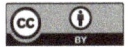

Copyright: © 2021 by the authors. Licensee MDPI, Basel, Switzerland. This article is an open access article distributed under the terms and conditions of the Creative Commons Attribution (CC BY) license (https://creativecommons.org/licenses/by/4.0/).

Abstract: Mental health issues among college students is a leading public health concern, which seems to have been exacerbating during the COVID-19 pandemic. While previous estimates related to psychological burden among college students are available, quantitative synthesis of available data still needs to be performed. Therefore, this meta-analysis endeavors to present collective evidence discussing the psychological impact of COVID-19 among college students. Bibliographical library databases, including Embase, Medline, CINAHL, Scopus, and PsycINFO, were systematically searched for relevant studies. Titles, abstracts, and full articles were screened, and two reviewers extracted data. Heterogeneity was assessed by I^2 statistic. The random-effects model was utilized to obtain the pooled estimates of psychological indicators among college students. Location, gender, level of severity, and quality scores were used as moderator variables for subgroup analyses. Funnel plot and Egger linear regression test was used to assess publication bias. Twenty-seven studies constituting 90,879 college students met the inclusion criteria. The results indicated 39.4% anxiety (95% CI: 28.6, 51.3; I^2 = 99.8%; p-value < 0.0001) and 31.2% depression (95% CI: 19.7, 45.6; I^2= 99.8%, p < 0.0001) among college students. The pooled prevalence of stress (26.0%), post-traumatic stress disorder (29.8%), and impaired sleep quality (50.5%) were also reported. College students bear a disproportionate burden of mental health problems worldwide, with females having higher anxiety and depression levels than males. This study''s findings underscore the need to develop appropriate public health interventions to address college students' emotional and psychosocial needs. The policies should be reflective of demographic and socioeconomic differentials.

Keywords: COVID-19; SARS-COV-2; anxiety; depression; stress; suicidal ideation; students

1. Introduction

By and large, college students generally experience several challenges, including starting new relationships, new life experiences, often new living situations, often an exploration of their sexual identities, usually academic pressures, need for time management, and sometimes balancing study, work, and personal life [1]. A study of college students investigating the psychological correlates found that the top concerns among this subgroup include pressure to succeed, educational performance, and post-college graduation plans [2,3]. These challenges make these students vulnerable to distress and associated negative sequelae such as depression, anxiety, insomnia, suicidal ideation, and adoption of maladaptive behaviors [1–3].

Mental health issues are alarmingly high among college students, particularly in the United States, with every eight in ten students experiencing frequent stress episodes in

2019 [4]. An eight-country study of 13,984 first-year college students under the World Health Organization's (WHO) World Mental Health Surveys found that the lifetime and annual prevalence of suicidal ideation in this group was 32.7% and 17.2%, respectively, which correspond to the high distress levels in the students' subgroup [5]. The likelihood of suicidal ideation increased twice following one or two traumatic events [1]. Among predictors of major depressive disorders, prior suicide plans/attempts, a history of childhood traumatic or stressful events, and family history contributed to college students' mental adversities [6]. These data are especially relevant in the context of U.S. college students, and the proportion of affected students may vary from country to country. Nonetheless, the mental health issues of college students emerge as a critical public health concern.

Mental health problems adversely affect numerous aspects of life. For college students, academic performance is the first to be affected. A Belgian study found that mental health problems have reduced college students' grade point average (GPA) by 0.2 to 0.3 points [7]. Depressive disorders among students are associated with cognitive impairments and real-world functioning [8]. The psychological impact among students extends further to the risk of adopting maladaptive behaviors, including binge drinking, smoking, substance abuse, overeating, risky sexual activities, dependence on social media, and sleep deprivation [8–10]. Stigma and embarrassment are also commonly associated with mental health problems among youth [11].

In December 2019, COVID-19 emerged as a public health threat and slowly became a worldwide pandemic, showing no curtailment signs while writing this manuscript [12]. COVID-19 has placed a considerable health burden and taxed the health care services around the world. Besides having a direct impact on physical health, it has had a severe toll on the psychological well-being of individuals due to fear, uncertainty, quarantine measures, lockdowns, social isolation, "infodemic" (or outpouring of news through various outlets, including social media), and so on [13–16]. In a study performed in India's post-phase two lockdown period, college students had higher stress and anxiety levels than the general population [17]. Many universities have closed in-person classes, vacated dormitories, and introduced online teaching, which has led to tremendous academic stress among students [18]. The adverse psychological outcomes have been compounded for students who are already facing higher levels of distress. Loneliness and insufficient perceived social support are detrimental to mental health [19], both of which have been accentuated in the COVID-19 pandemic. A mixed-methods study done at a public college in the United States found that 71% of the respondents had higher stress and anxiety with associated stressors of fear, worry, lack of concentration, and disruption in sleep during the COVID-19 pandemic [20]. College students who have recently moved away from their families are particularly susceptible to social deprivation and feelings of loneliness [21].

Further studies on students conducted in France, Ethiopia, China, and Malaysia also point at a high negative impact on college students' psychosocial health during the COVID-19 pandemic [22–24]. A study of college students in China found that the prevalence of post-traumatic stress disorder and depression rose to 2.7% and 9.0% during the COVID-19 pandemic [25]. Silva Junior et al. (2020) have published a protocol for conducting a systematic review on studying the psychological consequences of COVID-19 among young adults. However, no meta-analysis has yet been performed [26]. While the pooled estimates indicating the psychological impact of COVID-19 were reported for different population groups, including healthcare workers, the general population, and patients with pre-existing disorders, the collective evidence on college students' mental health still needs to be quantified [17,27–30]. Against this backdrop, this study attempts to conduct a meta-analysis of peer-reviewed published studies on the burden of psychological indicators among college students following the COVID-19 pandemic.

2. Materials and Methods

2.1. Protocol Registration

The preferred reporting items for systematic reviews and meta-analyses (PRISMA) guidelines were followed for this study [31]. This study's protocol was registered with the National Institute for Health Research (CRD42020203560), which serves as a prospective systematic review register. A detailed protocol can be found at https://www.crd.york.ac.uk/PROSPERO/display_record.php?RecordID=203560 (accessed on 16 February 2021).

2.2. Eligibility Criteria

We adapted the eligibility criteria used in the previous reports [27] to identify non-interventional and quantitative studies assessing the psychological impact of COVID-19 among college students. Studies were grouped according to the type of psychological morbidity observed, location (continent/country), quality score, and assessment method. Studies were included which met the following criteria: (1) use of the English language; (2) published from the inception of the pandemic to 27 July 2020; (3) utilized survey tools with good psychometric properties, and (4) full texts of the studies were available. Studies with the following characteristics were excluded: (1) Studies performed on populations other than students; (2) study designs utilizing descriptive, mixed-methods, qualitative approaches; (3) studies with unclear methodology or unvalidated survey tools; (4) studies using a language other than English; (5) studies conducted after 27 July 2020; (6) studies conducted among adolescents/students with pre-existing mental conditions, such as Attention Deficit Hyperactivity Disorder (ADHD); and (7) studies lacking the individual estimates for students.

2.3. Sources of Information

A search strategy was adapted from previous reports [27]. Library databases, including Medline (1946–2020), Embase (1974–2020), CINAHL (1937–2020), PsycINFO (1872–2020), and Scopus (1970–2020), were systematically searched.

2.4. Search Strategy

An experienced medical librarian (NS) designed the Medline search and then translated that search for use in the other databases [27]. When available, a search limit to the English language was applied, as was a publication date limit of 1 December 2019 to 27 July 2020. The search strings consisted of natural language terms and (when available) controlled vocabulary representing the concepts of "COVID-19" and "psychological outcomes." A detailed search strategy can be found in Appendix A, Box A1.

2.5. Selection Process

The search results were imported to Rayyan for the screening process. Two investigators (KB and MS) were involved in the screening of titles and abstracts to assess the articles' relevance with the research objective (Figure 1, Identification step). During the second level of screening, KB and MS independently evaluated all potential full-text articles (Figure 1, Screening step). In case of disagreements, the consensus among reviewers was built through discussions. The included publications addressed the psychological outcomes of COVID-19 among students. If multiple studies from the same authors were found, only the most recent manuscript was included in the analysis to avoid duplicate data bias. If any data discrepancies were noted in the articles, corresponding authors were contacted for verification.

2.6. Data Collection

Full-text articles were obtained for all studies that initially met the inclusion criteria. Two independent reviewers (KB and RB) abstracted all studies for potential inclusion and quality using a customized data abstraction form, resulting in an interrater agreement of 81%. Inconsistencies between reviewers were adjudicated by a third independent reviewer (MS). Information related to study authors, publication year, study location, gender distribution, number of subjects, type of survey tool with the cut-off criteria, and the proportion of subjects with positive psychological outcomes were collected in a spreadsheet. Data were reviewed twice to ensure accuracy. We also attempted to contact corresponding authors of the primary studies to verify the accuracy of data points (if needed).

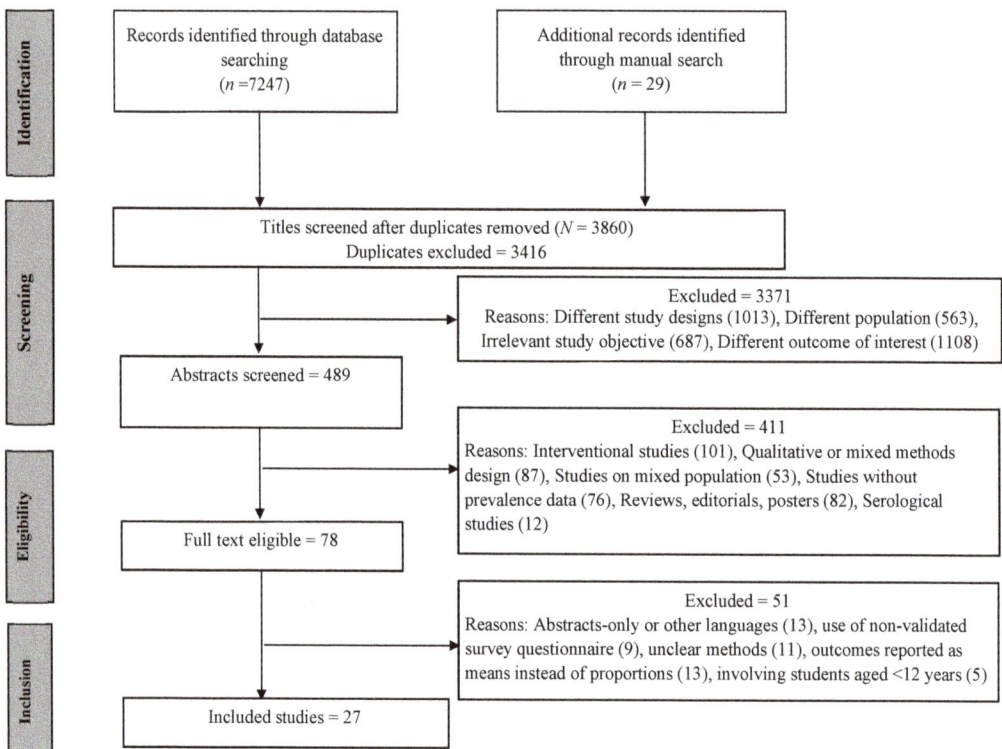

Figure 1. Preferred reporting items for systematic reviews and meta-analyses (PRISMA) flow diagram detailing all steps of screening with reasons for exclusion.

2.7. Assessment of Risk of Bias in Primary Studies

The National Institutes of Health (NIH) quality assessment tool was utilized for the risk of bias assessment. Two reviewers (KB and MS) independently evaluated the risk of bias and assigned the quality scores based on the tool's dictionary and guidelines (Appendix A, Table A1). The overall quality score was assigned according to the tool guidelines. In case of disagreements, the consensus among reviewers was built through discussions.

2.8. Measures of Effect and Data Analysis

The Comprehensive Meta-Analysis Package (CMA version 3.0, Englewood, NJ, USA) was utilized to compute the pooled estimates of psychological outcomes, including anxiety, depression, and other psychological indicators. The effect measure was the proportion of anxiety and depression events. The logit transformation of the proportions was used to meta-analyze the data. The Clopper–Pearson method was used to calculate exact confidence intervals for individual studies. Owing to methodologic differences across studies, a random-effects model was used to extract the pooled estimate [32]. Substantial heterogeneity was defined as $I^2 > 75\%$ [33]. Subgroup analyses by continent (Asia vs. other), country

(China vs. other), survey tool, study quality, gender, and levels of psychological outcomes were performed. Sensitivity analysis or leave-one-out analysis was also conducted to determine the impact of different weights assigned to each study on the final results. Funnel plot and Egger linear regression test statistics were utilized for publication bias [27,34]. *p*-values less than 0.05 were considered significant.

2.9. Assessment of Evidence

We assessed the certainty of the overall evidence based on the quality of individual studies and scientific rigor of the methodology used in each study. Two reviewers assessed the quality of the evidence and did not know each other's decision.

3. Results

3.1. Selection of the Dtudies

A total of 7276 relevant records were identified following systematic and manual search (Figure 1). The titles of the remaining 3860 records (after removing 3416 duplicates) were screened, of which only 489 articles advanced to the abstract screening step. Only 78 articles were found eligible (51 articles excluded) for the full-text screening, which later reduced to 27 articles for the final review or analysis. Reasons for exclusion are listed in Figure 1.

3.2. Characteristics of Included Studies

Twenty-seven studies (Appendix A, Table A2) [19,25,35–59] with a sample size of 90,879 students were finally assessed for generating pooled estimates. Eighteen studies were from Asia (14 from China, 1 from India, 1 from Israel, 1 from Jordan, and 1 from Saudi Arabia), seven were from Europe (two from Turkey, one from France, one from Greece, one from Italy, one from Russia and Belarus, and one from Albania), and two were from South and North America (one each). The median number of individuals across studies ranged from 66 to 44,447, with males constituting only 35% (n = 31,536) of the entire population. The remaining 50.4% (n = 45,824) of the sample constituted females. For the remaining 15% of the gender data, individual estimates for students were not provided.

3.3. Risk of Bias in the Included Studies

Eleven studies were assigned good quality scores [19,25,35,38,43,44,47,48,56,58,59] and sixteen studies were identified as of medium or fair quality [36,37,39–42,45,46,49–55,57] (Appendix A, Table A2). The kappa statistic (inter-rater agreement) was 89.5%.

3.4. Meta-Analysis

3.4.1. Anxiety

The pooled prevalence of anxiety in twenty studies [19,35,36,38–40,42–44,47,50–59] with a sample size 84,097 was 39.4% (95% CI: 28.6,51.3; I^2 = 99.8%; *p*-value < 0.0001; Table 1, Figure 2). Sub-analyses by additional categorical moderators, including gender, quality of study, continent, country, type of survey tool, and anxiety level were also conducted. Results of sub-analyses are given in Table 1.

3.4.2. Depression

The pooled prevalence of depression in fourteen studies [19,25,36,38,40,43,44,46–49,57–59] with a sample size 61,392 was 31.2% (95% CI: 19.7,45.6; I^2 = 99.8%, p < 0.0001, Table 2, Figure 3). Sub-analyses by additional categorical moderators, including gender, quality of study, continent, country, type of survey tool, and level of anxiety was also conducted (Table 2).

Table 1. Pooled estimates of anxiety by categorical moderator variables (subgroup analyses).

	Overall	Number of Studies	Proportion (%)	95% CI	I^2	p-Value	References
	Anxiety prevalence	20	34.4%	29.5,39.7	99.1%	<0.0001	[19,35,36,38–40,42–44,47,50–59]
			Subgroup Analysis				
Categories	Subgroups	Number of Studies	Proportion (%)	95% CI	I^2	p-Value	References
Quality	Good	9	29.3	16.8,45.8	99.8%	<0.0001	[19,35,38,43,44,47,56,58,59]
	Medium	11	48.4	33.0,64.1	99.6%	<0.0001	[36,39,40,42,50–55,57]
Continents	Asia	13	30.4	20.0,43.4	99.8%	<0.0001	[19,35,36,38,42,44,50,53,54,56–59]
	Other	7	57.5	38.6,74.4	98.8%	<0.0001	[39,40,43,47,51,52,55].
Countries	China	11	25.5	16.7,36.9	99.8%	<0.0001	[19,35,36,38,42,44,53,56–59]
	Other	9	58.7	44.0,72.0	98.7%	<0.0001	[39,40,43,47,50–52,54,55]
Assessment	GAD	8	33.0	18.1,52.3	99.4%	<0.0001	[35,38,43,44,53,54,57,59]
	Other	12	43.9	28.9,60.1	99.8%	<0.0001	[19,36,39,40,42,47,50–52,55,56,58]
Gender	Female	5	34.6	20.5,52.0	99.0%	<0.0001	[54,56–59]
	Male	5	22.9	36.3,52.5	98.3%	<0.0001	[54,56–59]
Level of Anxiety	Mild	7	73.7	63.8,81.7	96.9	<0.0001	[44,53–57,59]
	Moderate	7	23.1	16.2,31.8	97.7	<0.0001	[44,53–57,59]
	Severe	7	7.0	4.8,11.3	92.3	<0.0001	[44,53–57,59]

GAD: Generalized Anxiety Disorder.

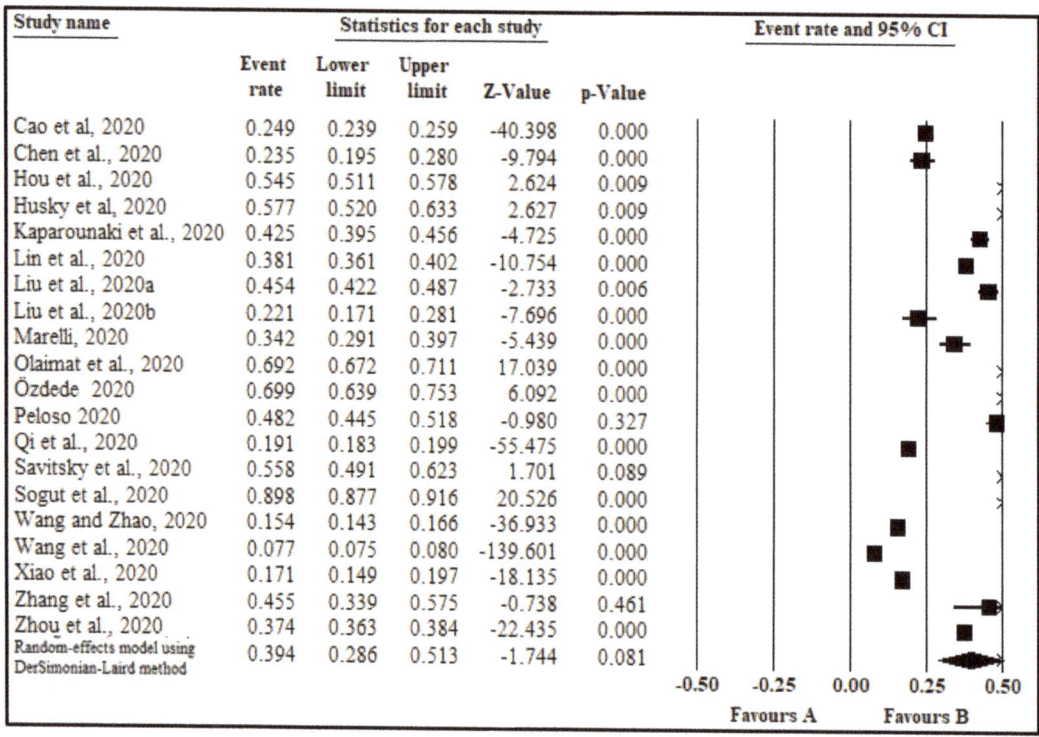

Figure 2. Forest plot showing pooled estimates of anxiety among students.

Table 2. Pooled estimates of depression by categorical moderator variables (subgroup analyses).

Overall		Number of Studies	Proportion (%)	95% CI	I^2	p-Value	References
Depression prevalence		14	31.2	19.7,45.6	99.8%	<0.0001	[19,25,36,38,40,43,44,46–49,57–59]
Subgroup Analysis							
Categories	Subgroups	Number of Studies	Proportion (%)	95% CI	I^2	p-Value	References
Quality	Good	9	29.7	16.4,47.7	99.8%	<0.0001	[19,25,38,43,44,47,48,58,59]
	Medium	5	34.0	15.6,59.0	99.3%	<0.0001	[36,40,46,49,57]
Continents	Asia	10	27.3	15.6,43.2	99.8%	<0.0001	[19,35,36,38,42,44,50,53,54,56–59]
	Other	4	42.2	19.3,69.1	99.3%	<0.0001	[40,43,47,48]
Countries	China	8	27.3	14.4,45.6	99.8%	<0.0001	[19,25,36,38,44,57–59]
	Other	6	36.8	18.8,59.5	99.1%	<0.0001	[40,43,46–49]
Assessment	PHQ	7	33.9	18.3,53.9	99.5%	<0.0001	[25,38,43,44,48,57,59]
	Other	7	28.7	14.9,48.0	99.6%	<0.0001	[19,36,40,46,47,49,58]
Gender	Female	5	32.4	20.0,44.8	96.4%	<0.0001	[44,49,57–59]
	Male	5	26.0	16.9,37.8	95.5%	<0.0001	[44,49,57–59]
Level of Anxiety	Mild	4	55.6	35.8,73.7	90.5%	<0.0001	[44,48,57,59]
	Moderate	4	30.4	17.5,47.5	97.4%	<0.0001	[44,48,57,59]
	Severe	4	16.1	8.2,29.3	96.9%	<0.0001	[44,48,57,59]

PHQ: Patient Health Questionnaire.

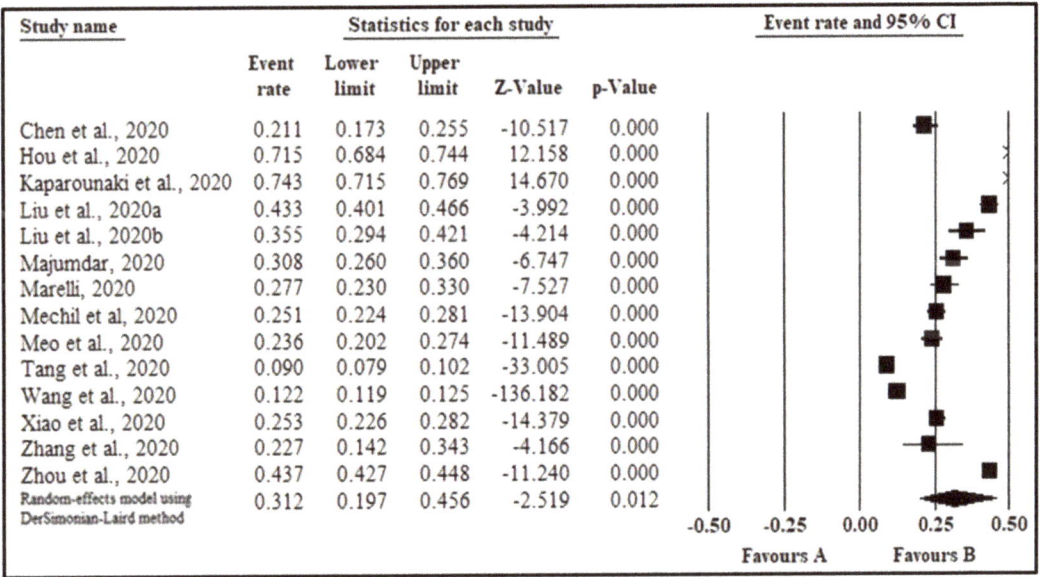

Figure 3. Forest plot indicating the pooled estimates of depression among students.

3.4.3. Other Psychological Outcomes

The pooled prevalence of stress in three studies [39,41,58] with a sample size of 1799 was 26.0% (95% CI: 7.7,59.5; I^2= 98.9%, p < 0.0001). Post-traumatic stress disorder (PTSD) in a sample of 4242 students across three studies [25,38,43] was 29.8% (95% CI:3.0, 85.4; I^2 = 99.8%, p < 0.001). The overall prevalence of impaired sleep quality among three studies [46,47,58] in a sample size of 698 was 50.5% (95% CI:23.9,76.8; I^2 = 97.6%;

$p < 0.001$). Suicidal ideation was assessed in only two studies [38,40] with rates of 31.3% and 63.3% respectively.

3.4.4. Publication Bias

Except anxiety ($p = 0.11$), P values of Egger test indicate insignificant publication bias for depression ($p = 0.17$), stress ($p = 0.68$), sleep disturbances ($p = 0.99$), and PTSD ($p = 0.78$).

3.4.5. Certainty of the Evidence

All primary studies were cross-sectional; therefore, the quality of the evidence would be moderate. However, most of the studies included in this analysis were of fair and good quality, which contributes to the certainty of the current meta-analysis evidence.

4. Discussion

The current metanalysis included 27 studies with a sufficiently large sample of ($N = 90,879$) college students to explore psychological dimensions during the pandemic. Prior studies and a few systematic review protocols [26] investigated the association between psychological health outcomes and COVID-19, but quantitative synthesis was lacking. To our knowledge, the current meta-analysis provides the first collective evidence of the negative psychological burden of COVID-19 on the mental health of college students. This evidence is critical to inform colleges, universities, and other educational institutions in designing interventions and policies to improve college students' mental health. Previous global evidence indicated that psychological morbidities were long-standing issues among college students even before the pandemic, with nearly 50% of mental issues starting at an early age of 14 years [60–62]. Globally, suicide remains among the leading causes of death among adolescents, which warrants the need to develop early interventions to address this population's mental health and emotional needs [62]. The consequences of not addressing these concerns during the early phases of life will be dire. A lack of early intervention may lead to psychological morbidities in later life phases [62]. Regarding the pandemic, it is important to intervene early to promote post-traumatic growth among students in existing and repairing phases of the pandemic. Our findings suggest a higher prevalence of anxiety (39.4%), depression (31.2%), and stress (26.0%) than those reported in the pre-pandemic period with 22.1% anxiety, 19.7% depression, and 13.4% stress [60–62]. Corollaries associated with COVID-19, including uncertainty and fear, exert an additional driving force to explain these rising trends [24]. The timeline to graduation, sudden transition to virtual learning, quality and logistics of internships, and post-graduation plans are all in uncertainty, causing significant distress among college students [24,52]. Association of other contributing factors, such as compliance to the new rules, propagation of ambiguous messages through media, and lack of scientific understanding, need to be explored fully to design a holistic public health approach to address mental health challenges among college students [60,62].

Additionally, young people like to socialize and indulge in parties and celebrations, which have been restricted in pandemic times, adding to their frustration levels [52,53,57]. Some students who receive counseling services have not been able to receive such support. Many students who work part-time jobs have lost their employment (voluntarily or employer initiated) during COVID-19, causing financial distress [24,52,53,57]. According to a study of 69,054 French students, nearly 42.8% of students reported having at least one negative mental health outcome; of those, only 12.4% sought assistance from healthcare professionals [24]. The stigma associated with seeking mental health support has been cited as a primary factor of underreported mental health issues among adolescents [62]. Among risk factors, the female gender is associated mainly with psychosocial health [24,53]. Females were twice as likely as males to experience mental health issues [24]. Our study found a significant gender gap in psychological morbidities. Females had significantly higher anxiety levels (34.6% vs. 22.9%) and depression (32.4% vs. 26.0%) than males. This finding was consistent with previous studies [24,63,64]. The gender differences may be attributed to a higher prevalence of pre-existing mental health conditions among females than males, complicated by introversion, higher sensitivity to traumatic events, and other factors, including hormonal imbalances and genetic vulnerability, and a higher mental health stigma among men [64–66]. Additional evidence reported that it is likely that mental health issues among men are underreported because of their tendency not to seek help from others [67].

We found a wider variation while making country comparisons. Anxiety and depression reported out of Asian countries were lower compared to other countries. Traditional close-knit family systems in Asia can be a protecting factor overriding one significant risk factor of social isolation, which has shown to contribute to increased risk of mental health issues [66]. Additionally, Asian countries, especially China and India, have traditional medicine with products and services widely available that are acceptable, affordable, and culturally appropriate. Most importantly, these have been adopted by the various Asian countries' health care systems [68]. However, the efficacy of traditional medicine has not been fully proven in counteracting mental health problems.

4.1. Strengths and Limitations

This meta-analysis is the first to assess the psychological impact of COVID-19 among students. It is urgent and essential to know the global scope of the issue. This population group is already facing a disproportionate burden of psychological morbidities even before the pandemic. This study also has some limitations. First, the self-reporting nature of the data collected by the studies in our meta-analysis might not be an accurate representation of the clinical diagnosis of the psychological illness. Second, sampling bias may exist because nearly 66.6% (18 out of 27) of the studies were conducted in Asia and predominantly China (51.8%; 14 out of 27). The larger pool of studies from China may presumably be due to the greater interest of the Chinese researchers in unfolding the epidemiology of COVID-19, as China was the first country to be affected by COVID-19. Other countries might have other research priorities prior to the pandemic inception, which occurred two months following the pandemic emergence in China. Third, all studies included in this meta-analysis were cross-sectional, which only account for prevailing circumstances, thereby lacking a longitudinal aspect to encounter temporality. Fourth, the studies included were only published in the English language, which might have introduced a language bias. Last, most of the studies included in this meta-analysis did not provide the year-wise, program (undergraduate/postgraduate), and type of course (e.g. STEM vs. non-STEM) stratifications of the students, which restricted our ability to determine differences in psychological morbidities among these groups. Future studies can be designed to account for differences in psychological outcomes across different groups of students to design a more targeted interventional approach.

4.2. Implications for Practice

This study advocates for designing and implementing appropriate interventions or programs to promote the mental health of students. The new policies and interventions will need to address gender differentials, such as designing tailored interventions for girls to address their specific needs. The use of telehealth has also been expanded in COVID-19, which can be used to offer remote counseling interventions across school or college campuses. Online implementation of mental health programs should be emphasized in lower or middle-income countries, which was reported to be a neglected field despite having good internet use [68]. Regular counseling centers for in-person visits across campuses with limited access to technology can also be beneficial. Besides, efforts should be directed towards increasing the quality of mental health services provided to the students. Mental health services provided by trained staff are improving. However, there are some gaps to be filled. According to the Association for College and College Counseling Center Directors (AUCCCD), comprising counseling directors of educational institutions from the United States, Canada, Europe, the Middle East, Asia, and Australia, one in five centers on their campus were reported to be lacking the optimum quality of mental health services [61,62]. The guided ways of stress management as implemented in certain universities in the US can be tailored towards a more comprehensive virtual delivery during the times of COVID-19. The American Council on Education advisory for the leadership ensures readiness of campuses for handling the increased burden on students' mental health. This involves regularly performing the needs assessment of college students from diverse backgrounds to design prospective policies and interventions. Healthy Minds Study or the American College Health Association-National College Health Assessment are examples that can be launched campus-wide to collect data for assessment and targeted intervention development.

5. Conclusions

College students bear a disproportionate burden of mental health problems worldwide, with females having higher anxiety and depression levels than males. This study's findings underscore the need to develop appropriate public health interventions to address adolescents' emotional, psychological, and social needs. The policies should be reflective of demographic and socioeconomic differentials.

Author Contributions: Conceptualization, analysis, screening, and investigations: K.B. and R.B.; Search strategy: N.S.; Methodology: K.B., M.S., and R.B.; Writing—original draft: K.B., R.B., T.P.S., M.S., and N.S.; Writing—review and editing: all authors. All authors have read and agreed to the published version of the manuscript.

Funding: No funding.

Institutional Review Board Statement: Not Applicable.

Informed Consent Statement: Not Applicable.

Data Availability Statement: Data are contained within the article or Appendix A.

Conflicts of Interest: The authors declare no conflict of interest.

Appendix A

Box A1. Detailed search strategy (executed 27 July 2020) for the identfication of records discussing the psychological impact of COVID-19 among college students

Database: Ovid MEDLINE(R) and Epub Ahead of Print, In-Process & Other Non-Indexed Citations and Daily <1946 to 27 July 2020> Search Strategy:
1   (2019nCoV or 2019-nCoV or coronavirus or coronavirinae or (corona adj3 (virinae or virus)) or "Corona virinae19" or "Corona virinae2019" or "corona virus19" or "corona virus2019" or Coronavirinae19 or Coronavirinae2019 or coronavirus19 or coronavirus2019 or covid19 or COVID-19 or SARS-CoV-2 or "Severe Acute Respiratory Syndrome Corona virus 2" or "Severe Acute Respiratory Syndrome Coronavirus 2").ti,ab,kw. [covid-19 keywords] (46270)   2   coronavirus/ or Coronavirus Infections/ [covid-19 MeSH] (19104)   3   or/1-2 [covid-19 set] (48733)   4   mental health/ or mental fatigue/ or Affective Symptoms/ or psychological distress/ [Mental health MeSH] (53257)   5   (emotional disturbanc* or affective symptom* or Alexithymia* or ((mental or psychological) adj3 (fatigue or health or status or distress or well-being)) or psychosocial).ti,ab,kw. [mental health keywords] (283768)   6   or/4-5 [mental health set] (305532)   7   Stress, Psychological/ or occupational stress/ or compassion fatigue/ or burnout, psychological/ or burnout, professional/ [stress MeSH] (131108)   8   (stress* or "adaptation syndrome" or (caregiver adj4 (burden or fatigue)) or "compassion fatigue" or "reality shock" or "social defeat").ti,ab,kw. [stress keywords] (842732)   9   or/7-8 [stress set] (897231)   10   Depression/ or anhedonia/ [depression MeSH] (119688)   11   (depression or depressed or anhedonia or dysphoria or dysthymia or melancholia or sadness).ti,ab,kw. [depression keywords] (404119)   12   or/10-11 [depression set] (436174)   13   anxiety/ or catastrophization/ [anxiety MeSH] (81955)   14   (anxiety or Catastrophiz* or hypervigilan* or nervousness).ti,ab,kw. [anxiety keywords] (195877)   15   or/13-14 [anxiety set] (218337)   16   "Sleep Initiation and Maintenance Disorders"/ [insomnia MeSH] (13134)   17   (drowsiness or dyssomnia* or hypersomnia* or insomnia* or parasomnia* or sleepless* or sleepwalk* or somnambul* or somnolen* or sopor or (sleep adj5 (disorder* or disturbance* or fragmented or debt or depriv* or walk*))).ti,ab,kw. [insomnia keywords] (77668)   18   or/16-17 [insomnia set] (80743)   19   or/6,9,12,15,18 [psychosocial outcomes set] (1621212)   20   and/3,19 [final set] (2483)   21   limit 20 to yr="2019 -Current" (2313)   22   limit 21 to english language (2221)

Table A1. Methodological quality assessment of included studies using the National Institutes of Health (NIH) tool.

Author/Year	Q1	Q2	Q3	Q4	Q5	Q6	Q7	Q8	Q9	Q10	Q11	Q12	Q13	Q14	Final Quality Score	Rating
Cao et al., 2020 [35]	Y	Y	Y	Y	NA	Y	N	N	Y	NA	Y	NA	NA	N	7	Good
Chen et al., 2020 [36]	Y	Y	N	N	NA	Y	N	N	Y	NA	Y	NA	NA	N	5	Fair
Gritsenko et al., 2020 [37]	Y	Y	N	N	NA	Y	N	N	Y	NA	Y	NA	NA	N	5	Fair
Hou et al., 2020 [38]	Y	Y	N	Y	NA	Y	Y	Y	Y	NA	N	NA	NA	N	7	Good
Husky et al., 2020 [39]	Y	Y	N	N	N	Y	N	N	Y	NA	Y	NA	NA	N	5	Fair
Kaparounaki et al., 2020 [40]	Y	Y	NR	N	NA	Y	N	N	Y	NA	NA	NA	NA	N	4	Fair
Li et al., 2020 [41]	Y	Y	Y	N	NA	Y	N	N	Y	NA	Y	NA	NA	N	6	Fair
Lin et al., 2020 [42]	Y	Y	NR	N	N	Y	Y	N	Y	NA	Y	NA	NA	N	6	Fair
Liu et al., 2020 [43]	Y	Y	Y	N	N	Y	N	N	Y	NA	Y	NA	NA	N	6	Fair
Liu et a., 2020 [44]	Y	Y	Y	Y	N	Y	N	N	Y	NA	Y	NA	NA	N	7	Good
Liu et al., 2020 [45]	Y	Y	NR	N	N	Y	N	Y	Y	NA	Y	NA	NA	N	6	Fair
Majumdar et al., 2020 [46]	Y	Y	N	N	N	Y	N	Y	NR	NA	Y	NA	NA	N	5	Fair

Author/Year	Q1	Q2	Q3	Q4	Q5	Q6	Q7	Q8	Q9	Q10	Q11	Q12	Q13	Q14	Final quality score	Rating
Marelli et al., 2020 [47]	Y	Y	N	N	Y	Y	Y	N	Y	NA	Y	NA	NA	N	7	Good
Mechil et al., 2020 [48]	Y	Y	NR	N	Y	Y	Y	N	Y	NA	Y	NA	NA	N	7	Good
Meo et al., 2020 [49]	Y	Y	Y	N	N	Y	N	N	Y	NA	Y	NA	NA	N	6	Fair
Olaimat et al., 2020 [50]	Y	Y	Y	N	N	Y	N	N	Y	NA	Y	NA	NA	N	6	Fair
Ozdede et al., 2020 [51]	Y	Y	Y	N	N	Y	N	N	Y	NA	Y	NA	NA	N	6	Fair
Peloso et al., 2020 [52]	Y	Y	Y	N	N	Y	Y	N	Y	NA	Y	NA	NA	N	6	Fair
Qi et al., 2020 [53]	Y	Y	N	N	N	Y	Y	N	Y	NA	Y	NA	NA	N	6	Fair
Savitsky et al., 2020 [54]	Y	Y	Y	N	N	Y	N	N	Y	NA	Y	NA	NA	N	6	Fair
Sogut et al., 2020 [55]	Y	Y	NR	N	N	Y	Y	N	Y	NA	Y	NA	NA	N	6	Fair
Tang et al., 2020 [25]	Y	Y	NR	Y	Y	Y	Y	N	Y	NA	Y	NA	NA	N	8	Good
Wang and Zhao et al., 2020 [56]	Y	Y	NR	N	Y	Y	Y	N	Y	NA	Y	NA	NA	N	7	Good

Table A1. Cont.

Author/Year	Q1	Q2	Q3	Q4	Q5	Q6	Q7	Q8	Q9	Q10	Q11	Q12	Q13	Q14	Final Quality Score	Rating
Wang et al., 2020 [19]	Y	Y	Y	N	N	Y	Y	N	Y	NA	Y	NA	NA	N	8	Good
Xiao et al., 2020 [57]	Y	Y	NR	Y	N	Y	Y	N	Y	NA	N	NA	NA	N	6	Fair
Zhang et al., 2020 [58]	Y	Y	NR	N	Y	Y	Y	N	Y	NA	Y	NA	NA	N	7	Good
Zhou et al., 2020 [59]	Y	Y	Y	N	Y	Y	Y	N	Y	NA	Y	NA	NA	N	8	Good

Y: Yes, b. N: No, c. NR: Not reported, d. NA: Not applicable; Q1. Clarity of research question; Q2. Detailed description of population; Q3. Participation rate of eligible participants (at least 50%); Q4. Clarity in the inclusion and exclusion criteria; Q5. Sample size justification, power description, or variance and effect estimates; Q6. Temporality of exposure and outcome; Q7. Sufficient timeframe; Q8. Levels of exposure; Q9. Frequency of exposure assessment; Q10. Description of independent variables; Q11. Description of dependent variables; Q12. Blinding; Q13. Loss to follow-up (response rate) after baseline 20% or less; Q14. Measurement of key potential confounding variables and statistical adjustment for their impact on the relationship between exposure(s) and outcome(s); Rating—Good, Fair or Poor: Good = (7–9 yes); fair = (4–6 yes).

Table A2. Data summarization of the included studies.

Author/Year [Reference #]	Sample Size	Quality Score	Country	Male (%)	Survey Tool	Outcomes (%) (n)	
						Anxiety	Depression
Cao et al., 2020 [35]	7143	7	China	30	GAD7	24.9 –1776	NA
Chen et al., 2020 [36]	383	5	China	NA	DSRS-C SCARED	23.5 –90	21.2 –81
Gritsenko et al., 2020 [37]	939	5	Russia and Belarus	19	FCV-19S	NA	NA
Hou et al., 2020 [38]	859	7	China	61	PHQ9 GAD7 IESR	54.5 –468	71.5 –614
Husky et al., 2020 [39]	291	5	France	25	World Mental Health International College Student Survey	57.7 –168	NA
Kaparounaki et al., 2020 [40]	1000	4	Greece	31	STAI CES-D RASS	42.5 –425	74.3 –743
Li et al., 2020 [41]	1442	6	China	NA	K6 IESR	NA	NA

Table A2. Cont.

Author/Year [Reference #]	Sample Size	Quality Score	Country	Male (%)	Survey Tool	Outcomes (%) (n) Anxiety	Outcomes (%) (n) Depression
Lin et al., 2020 [42]	2086	6	China	NA	STAI	38.1 –795	NA
Liu et al., 2020 [43]	898	6	USA	14	PHQ8 GAD7	45.4 –408	43.3 –389
Liu et al., 2020 [44]	217	7	China	41	PHQ9 GAD7	22.1 –48	35.5 –77
Liu et al., 2020 [45]	198	6	China	34	SSS	NA	NA

Author/Year	Sample Size	Quality Score	Country	Male (%)	Survey Tool	Outcomes (%) (n) Anxiety	Outcomes (%) (n) Depression
Majumdar et al., 2020 [46]	325	5	India	39	CES-D	NA	30.77 –100
Marelli et al., 2020 [47]	307	7	Italy	25	BAI BDI-II PSQI ISI	34.3 –105	27.8 –85
Mechili et al., 2020 [48]	863	7	Albania	11	PHQ9	NA	25.2 –217
Meo et al., 2020 [49]	530	6	Saudi Arabia	45	Stress Allied Queries	NA	23.6 –125
Olaimat et al., 2020 [50]	2083	6	Jordan	25	NA	69.2 –1441	NA
Özdede et al., 2020 [51]	249	6	Turkey	38	STAI	69.9 –174	NA
Peloso et al., 2020 [52]	704	6	Brazil (South America)	20	NA	48.2 –339	NA

Table A2. Cont.

Author/Year	Sample Size	Country	Male (%)	Survey Tool	Outcomes (%) (n) Anxiety	Outcomes (%) (n) Depression
Qi et al., 2020 [53]	9554	6	China	NA	GAD7	19 –1814	NA
Savitsky et al., 2020 [54]	215	6	Israel	12	GAD7	55.9 –120	NA
Sogut et al., 2020 [55]	972	6	Turkey	0	BAI	–873	NA
Tang et al., 2020 [25]	2485	8	China	39	PHQ9	NA	9 –224
Wang and Zhao, 2020 [56]	3611	7	China	40	SAS	–557	NA

Author/Year	Sample Size	Country	Male (%)	Survey Tool	Outcomes (%) (n) Anxiety	Outcomes (%) (n) Depression
Wang et al., 2020 [19]	44447	8	China	45	SAS CES-D	7.7 –3422	12.2 –5422
Xiao et al., 2020 [57]	933	6	China	30	GAD7 PHQ9	17.1 –160	25.3 –236
Zhang et al., 2020 [58]	66	7	China	38	DASS21 PSQI	–30	–15
Zhou et al., 2020 [59]	8079	8	China	46	PHQ-9 GAD-7	37.4 –3020	43.7 –3533

References

1. Liu, C.H.; Stevens, C.; Wong, S.H.M.; Yasui, M.; Chen, J.A. The prevalence and predictors of mental health diagnoses and suicide among U.S. college students: Implications for addressing disparities in service use. *Depress. Anxiety* **2019**, *36*, 8–17. [CrossRef] [PubMed]
2. Beiter, R.; Nash, R.; McCrady, M.; Rhoades, D.; Linscomb, M.; Clarahan, M.; Sammut, S. The prevalence and correlates of depression, anxiety, and stress in a sample of college students. *J. Affect. Disord.* **2015**, *173*, 90–96. [CrossRef] [PubMed]
3. Woodford, M.R.; Han, Y.; Craig, S.; Lim, C.; Matney, M.M. Discrimination and mental health among sexual minority college students: The type and form of discrimination does matter. *J. Gay Lesbian Ment. Health* **2014**, *18*, 142–163. [CrossRef]
4. Stress: An Epidemic among College Students. The American Institute of Stress Website. 2019. Available online: https://www.stress.org/stress-an-epidemic-among-college-students (accessed on 12 January 2021).
5. Mortier, P.; Auerbach, R.P.; Alonso, J.; Bantjes, J.; Benjet, C.; Cuijpers, P.; Ebert, D.D.; Green, J.G.; Hasking, P.; Nock, M.K.; et al. Suicidal thoughts and behaviors among First-Year college students: Results from the WMH-ICS Project. *J. Am. Acad. Child Adolesc. Psychiatry* **2018**, *57*, 263–273.e1. [CrossRef] [PubMed]
6. Ebert, D.D.; Buntrock, C.; Mortier, P.; Auerbach, R.; Weisel, K.K.; Kessler, R.C.; Cuijpers, P.; Green, J.G.; Kiekens, G.; Nock, M.K.; et al. Prediction of major depressive disorder onset in college students. *Depress. Anxiety* **2019**, *36*, 294–304. [CrossRef]
7. Bruffaerts, R.; Mortier, P.; Kiekens, G.; Auerbach, R.P.; Cuijpers, P.; Demyttenaere, K.; Green, J.G.; Nock, M.K.; Kessler, R.C. Mental health problems in college freshmen: Prevalence and academic functioning. *J. Affect. Disord.* **2018**, *225*, 97–103. [CrossRef] [PubMed]
8. Dhillon, S.; Videla-Nash, G.; Foussias, G.; Segal, Z.V.; Zakzanis, K.K. On the nature of objective and perceived cognitive impairments in depressive symptoms and real-world functioning in young adults. *Psychiatry Res.* **2020**, *287*, 112932. [CrossRef] [PubMed]
9. Kenney, S.R.; Lac, A.; Labrie, J.W.; Hummer, J.F.; Pham, A. Mental health, sleep quality, drinking motives, and alcohol-related consequences: A path-analytic model. *J. Stud. Alcohol. Drugs.* **2013**, *74*, 841–851. [CrossRef]
10. Malla, A.; Shah, J.; Iyer, S.; Boksa, P.; Joober, R.; Andersson, N.; Lal, S.; Fuhrer, R. Youth mental health should be a top priority for health care in Canada. *Can. J. Psychiatry* **2018**, *63*, 216–222. [CrossRef]
11. Gulliver, A.; Griffiths, K.M.; Christensen, H. Perceived barriers and facilitators to mental health help-seeking in young people: A systematic review. *BMC Psychiatry* **2010**, *10*, 113. [CrossRef]
12. World Health Organization. Coronavirus disease (COVID-19) Pandemic. 2020. Available online: https://www.who.int/emergencies/diseases/novel-coronavirus-2019 (accessed on 21 December 2020).
13. Balhara, Y.P.S.; Kattula, D.; Singh, S.; Chukkali, S.; Bhargava, R. Impact of lockdown following COVID-19 on the gaming behavior of college students. *Indian J. Public Health* **2020**, *64* (Supplement.), S172–S176. [CrossRef]
14. Dubey, S.; Biswas, P.; Ghosh, R.; Chatterjee, S.; Dubey, M.J.; Chatterjee, S.; Lahiri, D.; Lavie, C.J. Psychosocial impact of COVID-19. *Diabetes Metab. Syndr.* **2020**, *14*, 779–788. [CrossRef] [PubMed]
15. Khan, S.; Siddique, R.; Li, H.; Ali, A.; Shereen, M.A.; Bashir, N.; Xue, M. Impact of coronavirus outbreak on psychological health. *J. Glob. Health* **2020**, *10*, 010331. [CrossRef] [PubMed]
16. Li, H.Y.; Cao, H.; Leung, D.Y.P.; Mak, Y.W. The Psychological impacts of a COVID-19 outbreak on college Students in China: A Longitudinal Study. *Int. J. Environ. Res. Public Health* **2020**, *17*, 3933. [CrossRef]
17. Kaurani, P.; Batra, K.; Rathore-Hooja, H. Psychological impact of COVID-19 lockdown (Phase 2) among Indian general population: A cross-sectional analysis. *Int. J. Sci. Res.* **2020**, *9*, 51–56. [CrossRef]
18. Zhai, Y.; Du, X. Addressing collegiate mental health amid COVID-19 pandemic. *Psychiatry Res.* **2020**, *288*, 113003. [CrossRef] [PubMed]
19. Wang, Z.H.; Yang, H.L.; Yang, Y.Q.; Liu, D.; Li, Z.-H.; Zhang, X.-R.; Zhang, Y.-J.; Shen, D.; Chen, P.-L.; Song, W.-Q.; et al. Prevalence of anxiety and depression symptom, and the demands for psychological knowledge and interventions in college students during COVID-19 epidemic: A large cross-sectional study [published correction appears in J Affect Disord]. *J Affect Disord.* **2020**, *275*, 188–193. [CrossRef] [PubMed]
20. Son, C.; Hegde, S.; Smith, A.; Wang, X.; Sasangohar, F. Effects of COVID-19 on college students' mental health in the United States: Interview survey study. *J. Med. Internet Res.* **2020**, *22*, e21279. [CrossRef]
21. Orben, A.; Tomova, L.; Blakemore, S.J. The effects of social deprivation on adolescent development and mental health. *Lancet Child Adolesc. Health.* **2020**, *4*, 634–640. [CrossRef]
22. Aylie, N.S.; Mekonen, M.A.; Mekuria, R.M. The psychological impacts of COVID-19 pandemic among College students in Bench-Sheko Zone, South-west Ethiopia: A community-based cross-sectional study. *Psychol. Res. Behav. Manag.* **2020**, *13*, 813–821. [CrossRef]
23. Sundarasen, S.; Chinna, K.; Kamaludin, K.; Nurunnabi, M.; Baloch, G.M.; Khoshaim, H.B.; Hossain, S.F.A.; Sukayt, A. Psychological impact of COVID-19 and lockdown among College students in Malaysia: Implications and policy recommendations. *Int. J. Environ. Res. Public Health* **2020**, *17*, 6206. [CrossRef] [PubMed]
24. Wathelet, M.; Duhem, S.; Vaiva, G.; Baubet, T.; Habran, E.; Veerapa, E.; Debien, C.; Molenda, S.; Horn, M.; Grandgenèvre, P.; et al. Factors associated with mental health disorders among College students in France confined during the COVID-19 pandemic. *JAMA Netw. Open.* **2020**, *3*, e2025591. [CrossRef]

25. Tang, W.; Hu, T.; Hu, B.; Jin, C.; Wang, G.; Xie, C.; Chen, S.; Xu, J. Prevalence and correlates of PTSD and depressive symptoms one month after the outbreak of the COVID-19 epidemic in a sample of home-quarantined Chinese College students. *J. Affect. Disord.* **2020**, *274*, 1–7. [CrossRef] [PubMed]
26. Silva Junior, F.J.G.D.; Sales, J.C.E.S.; Monteiro, C.F.S.; Costa, A.P.C.; Campos, L.R.B.; Miranda, P.I.G.; Monteiro, T.A.D.S.; Lima, R.A.G.; Lopes-Junior, L.C. Impact of COVID-19 pandemic on mental health of young people and adults: A systematic review protocol of observational studies. *BMJ Open* **2020**, *10*, e039426. [CrossRef]
27. Batra, K.; Singh, T.P.; Sharma, M.; Batra, R.; Schvaneveldt, N. Investigating the Psychological impact of COVID-19 among healthcare workers: A Meta-Analysis. *Int. J. Environ. Res. Public Health* **2020**, *17*, 9096. [CrossRef]
28. Lakhan, R.; Agrawal, A.; Sharma, M. Prevalence of depression, anxiety, and stress during COVID-19 pandemic. *J. Neurosci. Rural Pract.* **2020**, *11*, 519–525. [CrossRef] [PubMed]
29. Luo, M.; Guo, L.; Yu, M.; Jiang, W.; Wang, H. The psychological and mental impact of coronavirus disease 2019 (COVID-19) on medical staff and general public-A systematic review and meta-analysis. *Psychiatry Res.* **2020**, *291*, 113190. [CrossRef]
30. Pappa, S.; Ntella, V.; Giannakas, T.; Giannakoulis, V.G.; Papoutsi, E.; Katsaounou, P. Prevalence of depression, anxiety, and insomnia among healthcare workers during the COVID-19 pandemic: A systematic review and meta-analysis. *Brain Behav. Immun.* **2020**, *88*, 901–907. [CrossRef]
31. Liberati, A.; Altman, D.G.; Tetzlaff, J.; Mulrow, C.; Gøtzsche, P.C.; Ioannidis, J.P.A.; Clarke, M.; Devereaux, P.J.; Kleijnen, J.; Moher, D. The PRISMA statement for reporting systematic reviews and meta-analyses of studies that evaluate healthcare interventions: Explanation and elaboration. *BMJ* **2009**, *339*, b2700. [CrossRef]
32. DerSimonian, R.; Laird, N. Meta-analysis in clinical trials. *Control. Clin. Trials* **1986**, *7*, 177–188. [CrossRef]
33. Higgins, J.P.; Green, S. Cochrane Handbook for Systematic Reviews of Interventions. John Wiley & Sons: Hoboken, NJ, USA, 2011.
34. Egger, M.; Smith, G.D.; Schneider, M.; Minder, C. Bias in meta-analysis detected by a simple, graphical test. *BMJ* **1997**, *315*, 629–634. [CrossRef] [PubMed]
35. Cao, W.; Fang, Z.; Hou, G.; Han, M.; Xu, X.; Dong, J.; Zheng, J. The psychological impact of the COVID-19 epidemic on college students in China. *Psychiatry Res.* **2020**, *287*, 112934. [CrossRef]
36. Chen, F.; Zheng, D.; Liu, J.; Gong, Y.; Guan, Z.; Lou, D. Depression and anxiety among adolescents during COVID-19: A cross-sectional study. *Brain Behav. Immun.* **2020**, *88*, 36–38. [CrossRef] [PubMed]
37. Gritsenko, V.; Skugarevsky, O.; Konstantinov, V.; Khamenka, N.; Marinova, T.; Reznik, A.; Isralowitz, R. COVID 19 Fear, Stress, Anxiety, and Substance Use Among Russian and Belarusian College Students [published online ahead of print, 2020 May 21]. *Int. J. Ment. Health Addict.* **2020**, 1–7. [CrossRef]
38. Hou, T.Y.; Mao, X.F.; Dong, W.; Cai, W.P.; Deng, G.H. Prevalence of and factors associated with mental health problems and suicidality among senior high school students in rural China during the COVID-19 outbreak. *Asian J. Psychiatr.* **2020**, *54*, 102305. [CrossRef]
39. Husky, M.M.; Kovess-Masfety, V.; Swendsen, J.D. Stress and anxiety among College students in France during COVID-19 mandatory confinement. *Compr. Psychiatry* **2020**, *102*, 152191. [CrossRef]
40. Kaparounaki, C.K.; Patsali, M.E.; Mousa, D.V.; Papadopoulou, E.V.K.; Papadopoulou, K.K.K.; Fountoulakis, K.N. College students' mental health amidst the COVID-19 quarantine in Greece. *Psychiatry Res.* **2020**, *290*, 113111. [CrossRef] [PubMed]
41. Li, Y.; Wang, Y.; Jiang, J.; Valdimarsdóttir, U.A.; Fall, K.; Fang, F.; Song, H.; Lu, D.; Zhang, W. Psychological distress among health professional students during the COVID-19 outbreak. *Psychol. Med.* **2020**, 1–3. [CrossRef] [PubMed]
42. Lin, Y.; Hu, Z.; Alias, H.; Wong, L.P. Influence of mass and social media on psychobehavioral responses among medical students during the downward trend of COVID-19 in Fujian, China: Cross-Sectional Study. *J. Med. Internet Res.* **2020**, *22*, e19982. [CrossRef]
43. Liu, C.H.; Zhang, E.; Wong, G.T.F.; Hyun, S.; Hahm, H.C. Factors associated with depression, anxiety, and PTSD symptomatology during the COVID-19 pandemic: Clinical implications for U.S. young adult mental health. *Psychiatry Res.* **2020**, *290*, 113172. [CrossRef]
44. Liu, J.; Zhu, Q.; Fan, W.; Makamure, J.; Zheng, C.; Wang, J. Online mental health survey in a medical college in China during the COVID-19 outbreak. *Front. Psychiatry* **2020**, *11*, 459. [CrossRef]
45. Liu, S.; Liu, Y.; Liu, Y. Somatic symptoms and concern regarding COVID-19 among Chinese college and primary school students: A cross-sectional survey. *Psychiatry Res.* **2020**, *289*, 113070. [CrossRef]
46. Majumdar, P.; Biswas, A.; Sahu, S. COVID-19 pandemic and lockdown: Cause of sleep disruption, depression, somatic pain, and increased screen exposure of office workers and students of India. *Chronobiol Int.* **2020**, *37*, 1191–1200. [CrossRef]
47. Marelli, S.; Castelnuovo, A.; Somma, A.; Castronovo, V.; Mombelli, S.; Bottoni, D.; Leitner, C.; Fossati, A.; Ferini-Strambi, L. Impact of COVID-19 lockdown on sleep quality in College students and administration staff. *J. Neurol.* **2020**, *268*, 8–15. [CrossRef]
48. Mechili, E.A.; Saliaj, A.; Kamberi, F.; Girvalaki, C.; Peto, E.; Patelarou, A.E.; Bucaj, J.; Patelarou, E. Is the mental health of young students and their family members affected during the quarantine period? Evidence from the COVID-19 pandemic in Albania. *J. Psychiatr. Ment. Health Nurs.* **2020**. [CrossRef]
49. Meo, S.A.; Abukhalaf, A.A.; Alomar, A.A.; Sattar, K.; Klonoff, D.C. COVID-19 pandemic: Impact of quarantine on medical students' mental well-being and learning behaviors. *Pak. J. Med. Sci.* **2020**, *36*, S43–S48. [CrossRef]
50. Olaimat, A.N.; Aolymat, I.; Elsahoryi, N.; Shahbaz, H.M.; Holley, R.A. Attitudes, anxiety, and behavioral practices regarding COVID-19 among College students in Jordan: A cross-sectional study. *Am. J. Trop. Med. Hyg.* **2020**, *103*, 1177–1183. [CrossRef]

51. Özdede, M.; Sahin, S.C. Views and anxiety levels of Turkish dental students during the COVID-19 pandemic. *J. Stomatol.* **2020**, *73*, 123–128. [CrossRef]
52. Peloso, R.M.; Ferruzzi, F.; Mori, A.A.; Camacho, D.P.; Franzin, L.C.D.S.; Teston, A.P.M.; Freitas, K.M.S. Notes from the field: Concerns of health-related higher education students in Brazil pertaining to distance learning during the Coronavirus pandemic. *Eval. Health Prof.* **2020**, *43*, 201–203. [CrossRef] [PubMed]
53. Qi, H.; Liu, R.; Chen, X.; Yuan, X.; Li, Y.; Huang, H.; Zheng, Y.; Wang, G. Prevalence of anxiety and associated factors for Chinese adolescents during the COVID-19 outbreak. *Psychiatry Clin. Neurosci.* **2020**, *74*, 555–557. [CrossRef] [PubMed]
54. Savitsky, B.; Findling, Y.; Ereli, A.; Hendel, T. Anxiety and coping strategies among nursing students during the covid-19 pandemic. *Nurse Educ. Pract.* **2020**, *46*, 102809. [CrossRef] [PubMed]
55. Sögüt, S.; Dolu, İ.; Cangöl, E. The relationship between COVID-19 knowledge levels and anxiety states of midwifery students during the outbreak: A cross-sectional web-based survey. *Perspect. Psychiatr. Care* **2021**, *57*, 246–252. [CrossRef] [PubMed]
56. Wang, C.; Zhao, H. The impact of COVID-19 on anxiety in Chinese College students. *Front. Psychol.* **2020**, *11*, 1–8. [CrossRef]
57. Xiao, H.; Shu, W.; Li, M.; Li, Z.; Tao, F.; Wu, X.; Yu, Y.; Meng, H.; Vermund, S.H.; Hu, Y. Social Distancing among medical students during the 2019 Coronavirus disease pandemic in China: Disease awareness, anxiety disorder, depression, and behavioral activities. *Int. J. Environ. Res. Public Health* **2020**, *17*, 5047. [CrossRef]
58. Zhang, Y.; Zhang, H.; Ma, X.; Di, Q. Mental health problems during the COVID-19 pandemics and the mitigation effects of exercise: A longitudinal study of college students in China. *Int. J. Environ. Res. Public Health* **2020**, *17*, 3722. [CrossRef]
59. Zhou, S.J.; Zhang, L.G.; Wang, L.L.; Guo, Z.-C.; Wang, J.-Q.; Chen, J.-C.; Liu, M.; Chen, X.; Chen, J.-X. Prevalence and sociodemographic correlates of psychological health problems in Chinese adolescents during the outbreak of COVID-19. *Eur. Child Adolesc. Psychiatry* **2020**, *29*, 749–758. [CrossRef]
60. American Council on Education. Mental Health, Strategies for Leaders to Support Campus Well-Being. 2019. Available online: https://www.acenet.edu/Documents/Mental-Health-Higher-Education-Covid-19.pdf (accessed on 1 January 2021).
61. College Students' Mental Health Is a Growing Concern, Survey Finds. Monitor on Psychology. American Psychological Association Website. 2013. Available online: http://www.apa.org/monitor/2013/06/college-students (accessed on 1 January 2021).
62. World Health Organization. Adolescent Mental Health. 2020. Available online: https://www.who.int/news-room/fact-sheets/detail/adolescent-mental-health (accessed on 25 January 2020).
63. Ozdin, S.; Ozdin, S.B. Levels and predictors of anxiety, depression and health anxiety during COVID-19 pandemic in Turkish society: The importance of gender. *Int. J. Soc. Psychiatry* **2020**, *66*, 504–511. [CrossRef]
64. Wenjun, G.; Siqing, P.; Xinqiao, L. Gender differences in depression, anxiety, and stress among college students: A longitudinal study from China. *J. Affect. Disord.* **2020**, *263*, 292–300. [CrossRef]
65. Chaplin, T.M.; Hong, K.; Bergquist, K.; Sinha, R. Gender differences in response to emotional stress: An assessment across subjective, behavioral, and physiological domains and relations to alcohol craving. *Alcohol. Clin. Exp. Res.* **2008**, *32*, 1242–1250. [CrossRef]
66. Baldry, A.C.; Farrington, D. Protective Factors as Moderators of Risk Factors in Adolescence Bullying. *Soc. Psychol. Educ.* **2005**, *8*, 263–284. [CrossRef]
67. Rasmussen, M.L.; Hjelmeland, H.; Dieserud, G. Barriers toward help-seeking among young men prior to suicide. *Death Stud.* **2018**, *42*, 96–103. [CrossRef] [PubMed]
68. Cianconi, P.; Lesmana, C.B.J.; Ventriglio, A.; Janiri, L. Mental health issues among indigenous communities and the role of traditional medicine. *Int. J. Soc. Psychiatry* **2019**, *65*, 289–299. [CrossRef] [PubMed]

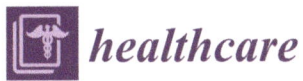

Article

The Psychological Symptoms of College Student in China during the Lockdown of COVID-19 Epidemic

Yin Li, Linbo Qin, Yaobin Shi and Jun Han *

College of Resources and Environment Engineering, Wuhan University of Science and Technology, Wuhan 430081, China; liyin@wust.edu.cn (Y.L.); qinlinbo@wust.edu.cn (L.Q.); shiyaobin@wust.edu.cn (Y.S.)
* Correspondence: hanjun@wust.edu.cn; Tel.:+86-27-6886-2880

Abstract: The COVID-19 epidemic has had a huge impact on the mental state of human beings due to its high infection and fatality rates in early 2020. In this paper, a cross-sectional online survey was designed to understand the mental state of college students in a university located in Wuhan city during the lockdown. Out of 1168 respondents, above 50% participants had obvious fear and anxiety symptoms; anxiety and fear were 61.64% and 58.39%, respectively. Conformity (49.49%), invulnerability (26.11%), insensitivity (21.49%) and rebelliousness (12.41%) symptoms also appeared. Meanwhile, it was revealed that the senior students experienced more anxiety than the freshmen. Moreover, it was found that the psychological symptoms (except for the insensitivity symptom) had no significant difference in gender, residence and annual household income after the one-way analysis of variance.

Keywords: psychological symptom; college student; COVID-19; lockdown

Citation: Li, Y.; Qin, L.; Shi, Y.; Han, J. The Psychological Symptoms of College Student in China during the Lockdown of COVID-19 Epidemic. *Healthcare* **2021**, *9*, 447. https://doi.org/10.3390/healthcare9040447

Academic Editors: Manoj Sharma and Kavita Batra

Received: 31 March 2021
Accepted: 9 April 2021
Published: 11 April 2021

Publisher's Note: MDPI stays neutral with regard to jurisdictional claims in published maps and institutional affiliations.

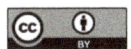

Copyright: © 2021 by the authors. Licensee MDPI, Basel, Switzerland. This article is an open access article distributed under the terms and conditions of the Creative Commons Attribution (CC BY) license (https://creativecommons.org/licenses/by/4.0/).

1. Introduction

In December 2019, COVID-19 first broke out in Wuhan city [1]. The virus could be spread by a person-to-person pattern including direct transmission, inhalation transmission and contact transmission. Afterwards, the virus quickly spread to China and the world [2]. Hence, COVID-19 was defined as a public health emergency of international concern on 30 January 2020 by the World Health Organization (WHO) and declared a pandemic on 12 March 2020 [3]. Up to 5 December 2020, there had been over 66 million reported confirmed cases of COVID-19 and 1.5 million deaths [4]. Wuhan city in the Hubei Province firstly implemented a Level 1 response to the public health emergency and a lockdown on 23 January 2020 due to the high fatality rate [1]. All public traffic was stopped and the movement of individuals was restricted. Most of the people, except for those involved in epidemic prevention and control, the police and few workers of necessary industries, were required to stay at home [5,6]. After Wuhan city, the government of all provinces in China implemented a Level 1 response to the public health emergency on 29 January 2020 [7]. Hence, all campuses of the universities in China were mandated to be closed in the spring of 2020 and the college students were required to stay at home and have their courses online to complete their academic study plan [8]. The long time of the lockdown caused people to get information, including a lot of fake news, from the media or the internet, which inevitably led to a stress response [9]. The transmission routes, origin and treatments of COVID-19 were not clearly understood at the early epidemic stage and the individual was only isolated in the home. Social interaction, physical activities and entertainment were prohibited and the normal living style was changed [10]. Meanwhile, surfing time increased and sleep and diets were irregular [11]. Thus, the long lockdown caused severe psychological symptoms such as anxiety, depression, insomnia and fear to the people isolated at home [12]. Qiu et al. carried out a survey and received 52,730 valid responses from 36 provinces as well as Hong Kong, Macau and Taiwan on 10 February 2020; they reported that 35% of the population in China experienced psychological distress during the COVID-19 epidemic [13]. A total of 1210 respondents from 194 cities in China took part in the survey within the first two weeks of the COVID-19 outbreak and the results of Wang et al. demonstrated that 28.8% of respondents had an anxious symptom of a moderate to severe level and 16.5% experienced moderate to severe depression symptoms [14]. Mazza et al. claimed that females exhibited a greater level of distress than males and had a higher level of anxiety. In addition, the respondents of the age of 18–30 and above 60 years were easier to be affected by distress than those with an age range of 30–60 [15]. College students are in the late adolescence stage with a high neurodevelopmental risk. Moreover, the supervision or attention from parents was significantly decreased [16] and college students were more vulnerable than the adults [12]. It was found that 7.7% of students were depressive, which was higher than that of the general population during the COVID-19 pandemic [17]. Anxiety, depression, sleep difficulties and stress were regarded as the main manifestations of the psychological symptoms in the disaster [18,19]. Wang et al. reported that the psychological symptoms for college students were moderate to severe anxiety (28.8%), depression (16.5%) and stress (8.1%) [20]. Fu et al. investigated the influence of variables such as sex, age, grade, place of residence and parent's education level on the anxiety of college students and claimed that the anxiety level of the students in the rural regions was higher than that of the urban regions and that the female students experienced more anxiety than the male students due to their biology [21].

In this paper, a cross-sectional online survey was designed to acquire the mental state of college students in a university of science and technology located in Wuhan city during the lockdown and the impact of the residence region (urban or rural), grade, gender and annual household income on the psychological symptoms was assessed. The survey results will help the office of student affairs to understand the mental state of the students. Based on previous publications, it was hypothesized that:

Hypothesis 1. *There is a significant difference of psychological symptoms with regard to the gender.*

Hypothesis 2. *There is a significant difference of psychological symptoms with regard to the residence.*

Hypothesis 3. *There is a significant difference of psychological symptoms with regard to the annual household income.*

2. Materials and Methods

The survey was designed according to a study conducted in a Chinese university [22], the Generalized Anxiety Disorder 7-Item Scale (GAD-7) [23] and the guiding principles of emergent psychological crisis intervention in COVID-19 [24]. Information such as age, gender, grade, health state, residence, annual household income and grade were collected using single item measures. Anxiety was obtained according to GAD-7 and Cronbach's alpha coefficient was 0.901. Invulnerability, conformity, insensitivity, rebelliousness and bravado were measured by a Likert-type scale of 1–4; "1 = Never or very rare", "2 = Sometimes", "3 = Often" and "4 = Very often or always". The risk level of the living region was decided according to the data from the National Health Commission of the People's Republic of China (a high risk region $\geq$ 50 confirmed cases in two weeks; the moderate risk region had < 50 confirmed cases and had new confirmed cases in two weeks; the mild risk region had no new confirmed case in two weeks). The cross-sectional survey was carried out from 1 April to 1 June 2020. The Questionnaire Star (https://www.wjx.cn, accessed on 30 June 2020) was used as the platform of this survey. The participants were recruited from the Wuhan University of Science and Technology (WUST) and the website of the survey was shared in WeChat or a QQ group of the students of WUST. Before the survey, an electronic informed consent was signed online. The participants were informed that the survey was anonymous and they could reject the survey for any reason. The study was approved by the Ethics Committee of Wuhan University of Science and Technology (protocol code 20200407, 4 February 2021). All data were analyzed by SPSS software and a one-way analysis of variance was applied to assess the significance of each factor.

3. Results

3.1. Characteristics of Participants

A total of 1168 students completed the survey (1237 students were informed and the valid rate was 94.4%). The age of the participants was 17–25; the numbers of freshmen, sophomores, juniors, seniors and graduate students were 397, 328, 102, 68 and 273, respectively. Of the respondents, 34.93% were female and 65.07% were male. A total of 599 lived in an urban region and 569 lived in a rural region. The annual household incomes were above 0.8 million (0.17%), 0.4–0.8 million (1.71%), 0.2–0.4 million (11.39%) and below 0.2 million (86.73%). About 99.66% participants were healthy and 0.34% were exposed, and no suspicion or infected existed. The number of participants who lived in the low risk regions was 385 (32.96%); those in the middle risk regions and the high risk regions were 681 (58.30%) and 102 (8.73%), respectively. The demographic characteristics of participants is summarized in Table 1.

Table 1. Demographic characteristics of participants ($n = 1168$).

Characteristics		Frequency
Gender	Male	408 (34.93%)
	Female	760 (65.07%)
Grade	Freshmen	397 (33.99%)
	Sophomore	328 (28.08%)
	Junior	102 (8.73%)
	Senior	68 (5.82%)
	Graduate student	273 (23.37%)
Residence	Rural	569 (48.72%)
	Urban	599 (51.28%)
Annual household income (RMB million)	>0.8	2 (0.17%)
	0.4–0.8	20 (1.71%)
	0.2–0.4	133 (11.39%)
	<0.2	1013 (86.73%)
Health state	Regular	1164 (99.66%)
	Exposed	4 (0.34%)
	Suspicion	0 (0.00%)
	Infected	0 (0.00%)
Risk level of living region	Low	385 (32.96%)
	Middle	681 (58.30%)
	High	102 (8.73%)

3.2. Psychological Symptoms of College Students during the Epidemic

Table 2 presents that most of the respondents had symptoms of fear and anxiety. A total of 58.39% participants experienced fear due to the high contagion level of COVID-19 and the mild, moderate and severe symptoms were 49.14%, 8.22% and 1.03%, respectively. At the same time, about 62.64% students had anxiety symptoms during the epidemic; moderate and severe anxiety were 0.02% and 6.51%, respectively.

3.3. Distribution of Anxiety by the Grade of College Students

It can observe from Table 3 that the high grade students had higher levels of anxiety than that of the freshmen and the percentage of freshmen, sophomores, juniors, seniors and graduate students who had fear symptoms were 53.15%, 61.59%, 58.82%, 60.29% and 61.54%, respectively.

Table 2. Psychological symptoms of college students during the COVID-19 epidemic.

Psychological Symptoms	Normal	Mild	Moderate	Severe
Fear	41.61%	49.14%	8.22%	1.03%
Anxiety	38.36%	54.02%	0.00%	6.51%
Invulnerability	73.89%	22.86%	2.23%	1.03%
Conformity	50.51%	40.5%	8.3%	0.68%
Bravado	88.01%	11.04%	0.77%	0.17%
Rebelliousness	87.59%	10.36%	1.71%	0.34%
Insensitivity	78.51%	18.84%	2.05%	0.6%

Table 3. Distribution of anxiety by the grade.

Level of Anxiety	Freshman	Sophomore	Junior	Senior	Graduate	Total Number
Normal	46.85%	38.41%	41.18%	39.71%	38.46%	486
Mild	44.33%	50.61%	51.96%	52.94%	52.38%	574
Moderate	7.56%	9.76%	4.90%	5.88%	9.16%	96
Severe	1.26%	1.22%	1.96%	1.47%	0.00%	12

3.4. Analysis of the Significance of Factors

A one-way within subject analysis of variance (ANOVA) was applied to assess the significance of each factor such as the gender, residence and annual household income, as shown in Tables 4–6. Table 4 demonstrates that the F values of the ANOVA were below 3.0 and the *p* values were above 0.05. Hence, it could be said that there was no difference in regard to the residence. Thus, Hypothesis 1 was not supported.

Table 4. The difference in psychological symptoms across the residences.

Variance	Residence (Mean ± SD)		F	p
	Urban (*n* = 599)	Rural (*n* = 569)		
Invulnerability	1.31 ± 0.58	1.30 ± 0.54	0.167	0.683
Conformity	1.58 ± 0.67	1.60 ± 0.67	0.146	0.703
Fear	1.68 ± 0.68	1.70 ± 0.65	0.218	0.641
Bravado	1.15 ± 0.41	1.11 ± 0.33	2.728	0.099
Rebelliousness	1.15 ± 0.46	1.14 ± 0.39	0.098	0.754
Insensitivity	1.26 ± 0.53	1.24 ± 0.49	0.436	0.509
Anxiety	2.32 ± 0.65	2.33 ± 0.64	0.071	0.790

F, test statistic; *p*, probability value.

Table 5. The impact of the risk level of the residence on anxiety.

Risk Level of Residence	Normal	Mild and Moderate	Severe	Total
High	25 (24.51%)	64 (62.75%)	13 (12.75%)	102 (8.73%)
Medium	255 (37.44%)	381 (55.95%)	45 (8.29%)	681 (58.30%)
Low	168 (43.64%)	186 (48.31%)	31 (8.05%)	385 (32.96%)

Table 6. The impact of the risk level of the residence on fear.

Risk Level of Residence	Normal	Mild	Moderate	Severe	Total
High	32 (31.37%)	51 (50.00%)	16 (15.69%)	3 (2.94%)	102 (8.73%)
Medium	253 (37.15%)	366 (53.74%)	56 (8.22%)	6 (0.88%)	681 (58.30%)
Low	201 (52.21%)	157 (40.78%)	24 (6.23%)	3 (0.78%)	385 (32.96%)

The impact of the risk level of the residence on the anxiety variation of participants is demonstrated in Table 5. It was found that 8.73% lived in a high risk level region;

58.30% and 32.96% were in the regions of medium and low risk levels. At the same time, the participants who lived in the medium and high risk level regions had greater anxiety than those of the low risk level regions. In addition, most of the participants appeared in the mild level of anxiety in this study.

Similar to the case of anxiety, the participants located in the safer regions experienced less fear, as shown in Table 6. The fear level of most of the participants was normal and mild. The safer areas had fewer restrictions and the participants could have more social interactions, physical activities and supplies, which was of benefit for good emotions.

According to Table 7, the F values of all psychological symptoms were below 3.0 and the p values were also above 0.05. Hence, it can be said that there was no obvious difference in regard to the gender so Hypothesis 2 was not supported.

Table 7. The difference in psychological symptoms across the genders.

Variance	Gender (Mean ± SD)		F	p
	Male(n = 760)	Female (n = 408)		
Invulnerability	1.40 ± 0.50	1.20 ± 0.41	2.400	0.128
Conformity	1.60 ± 0.75	1.63 ± 0.56	0.032	0.858
Fear	1.60 ± 0.60	1.77 ± 0.73	0.722	0.400
Bravado	1.15 ± 0.49	1.03 ± 0.18	1.421	0.239
Rebelliousness	1.10 ± 0.31	1.03 ± 0.18	0.925	0.341
Insensitivity	1.25 ± 0.44	1.23 ± 0.50	0.014	0.905
Anxiety	1.95 ± 0.60	2.17 ± 0.70	1.281	0.263

F, test statistic; p, probability value.

Table 8 demonstrates that there were no significant differences in invulnerability, conformity, fear, bravado, rebelliousness and anxiety in regard to the annual household income so Hypothesis 3 was not supported. However, the economical level of the family had an obvious influence on insensitivity during the epidemic period (F = 3.668, p = 0.033). The students with a medium annual household income had a high level of psychological symptoms such as invulnerability, conformity, fear, rebelliousness and insensitivity and the participants who had the highest annual household income had the highest level of anxiety.

Table 8. The difference in psychological symptoms across the annual household income.

Variance	Annual Household Income (RMB Million) (Mean ± SD)			F	p
	<0.2 (n = 1013)	0.2–0.4 (n = 133)	>0.4 (n = 22)		
Invulnerability	1.26 ± 0.44	1.38 ± 0.52	1.33 ± 0.58	0.241	0.787
Conformity	1.64 ± 0.63	1.75 ± 0.71	1.00 ± 0.00	1.661	0.201
Fear	1.72 ± 0.69	1.75 ± 0.71	1.33 ± 0.58	0.464	0.631
Bravado	1.08 ± 0.35	1.13 ± 0.35	1.00 ± 0.00	0.149	0.862
Rebelliousness	1.05 ± 0.22	1.13 ± 0.35	1.00 ± 0.00	0.403	0.670
Insensitivity	1.18 ± 0.39	1.63 ± 0.74	1.00 ± 0.00	3.668	0.033 *
Anxiety	2.08 ± 0.70	1.88 ± 0.35	2.67 ± 0.58	1.584	0.216

F, test statistic; p, probability value; * p < 0.05.

4. Discussions

In this survey, over half of all college students surveyed had psychological symptoms of fear and anxiety during the epidemic of COVID-19. In the early epidemic stage, the origin, transmission routes and suitable medicines were unknown. A lot of negative information and rumors about the virus emerged in the media or on the internet and governments had no time to debunk them. At the same time, college students were isolated in the home and spent a lot of time browsing the internet; thus, a greater number of negative psychological symptoms appeared [25]. College students are in the later stage of adolescence and their mental states can be more easily affected by the information from the internet or media [26]. Thus, the college students surveyed suffered from fear, anxiety, invulnerability, conformity, bravado, rebelliousness and insensitivity symptoms.

In this survey, 62.64% students had anxiety symptoms during the epidemic. Batra et al. assessed the psychological impact of COVID-19 among college students and found that the prevalence of anxiety in China was 25.5% compared with 58.7% in other regions [27]. The government strengthened the management of information released, the frequency of news release conferences increased and information or knowledge acquisition methods were also added. Thus, college students could know more information about COVID-19 and the cognition of COVID-19 was rebuilt. The level of the psychological symptoms appearing in college students gradually decreased [26].

In addition, the high grade students experienced more anxiety. The emotion variation was related to the worry of being infected, social support, income and academic delay [28]. The freshmen would not consider the graduation, employment and practice course [21], which would relieve part of the stress and anxiety [29]. Moreover, the higher grade students had greater academic pressure [21].

According to the results of Li et al., the risk level of the community had a linear relationship with the psychological symptoms of the residents (Severe $\geq$ 10,000 confirmed cases: Hubei province; Moderate = 1000–9999 confirmed cases: Guangdong, Henan, Hunan and Zhejiang provinces; Mild $\leq$ 1000 confirmed cases: all other provinces) [30]. Budimir et al. also thought that the risk level of the epidemic had a significant influence on mental health, e.g., depression, anxiety and insomnia [31]. In this survey, it was revealed that about 0.6% respondents had infected relatives, which had a negative effect on the emotional state of the students. However, Moghanibashi-Mansourieh claimed that belief was rebuilt after the relatives recovered from COVID-19 and the infected relatives had a positive influence on anxiety and stress reduction [32].

This survey revealed that there were no significant differences in gender, residence and annual household income and all hypotheses were not supported although there were significant differences of economy, infrastructure and policy of the central government between the rural and urban regions in China. In general, the economic situation in the rural regions was usually lower than in the urban region. At the same time, college students had to complete their study online and the internet in the rural regions was worse than in the urban regions [33]. Moreover, the urban regions had more hospitals and the patients could be promptly treated [28]. Food and medical supplies were also preferentially provided. However, rural regions usually have a low population density and the risk level was lower than that of urban regions. Hence, the limits of COVID-19 prevention in urban regions were stricter than those of the rural regions. Thus, there was no significant difference in the psychological symptoms with regard to the residence.

Insensitivity symptoms seemed to have a significant difference in the annual household income. The participants with a 0.2–0.4 Chinese Yuan (RMB) million annual household income had the highest level of insensitivity symptoms due to the middle-class family having no financial pressures. Rossell et al. reported that people under economic stress experience more negative emotions [34]. At the same time, the parents of the middle-class families had more time to accompany the children. The participants who had the highest household income had the highest anxiety because they were worried about their business.

Although females were more sensitive and emotional to the environment due to biological factors and females experienced greater anxiety and fear in the disaster [35], the present study also discovered that both female and male college students had similar negative psychological symptoms during the epidemic of COVID-19. This conclusion was consistent with previous studies [21,28].

In general, half of the participants had negative psychological symptoms. Suitable intervening methods or strategies such as online psychological counseling and online mental health education courses as well as opportunities for talking with classmates, friends or teachers should be provided, which could be useful for building a positive attitude and effectively reducing the stress or psychological symptoms. Social support was also important in maintaining the psychology of college students. In addition, the psychological resilience of college students played an important role in safeguarding their mental health [12].

Shorter studying hours, a reduced workload, keeping enough sleep time and regular eating of healthy food were should be considered to improve the resilient mentality [36].

5. Limitation

This study had a few limitations, which limited the application of this finding in other epidemics. Firstly, the study had a limited response of 1168 and all respondents came from one university located in Wuhan city. The generalizability of this finding was insufficient. Secondly, this study was undertaken between April and June, which was the medium stage of COVID-19; the views could not represent the final view such as the influence of infected relatives on the psychological symptoms of students. A secondary survey was necessary and the dynamic variations of the psychological symptoms should be tracked. Thirdly, the respondents were not equally distributed with regard to gender, grade and residence. Lastly, all data from the survey were obtained by self-reporting.

Although there were a few shortcomings, this study gave the psychological symptoms of college students in the COVID-19 epidemic, which was useful for choosing a suitable method of psychological intervention.

6. Future Direction

This survey investigated the dependence of psychological symptoms such as fear, anxiety, conformity, invulnerability, insensitivity and rebelliousness on the gender, residence and annual household income during the epidemic of COVID-19. A longitudinal study of the psychological symptoms during and after the epidemic is necessary and the severity of psychological symptoms can be understood. In addition, the relationship between psychological symptoms and academic study also should be considered. Lastly, it is also worth considering the influence of the suggested intervention methods on psychological symptoms.

7. Conclusions

In general, all members of society have had a huge stress due to the high fatality rate of COVID-19. Especially for relatives or friends who were infected by or exposed to COVID-19, stress levels sharply increased. Thus, the body shows stress responses such as the variation of emotions, biology, behavior and cognition. In this study, it was revealed that half of the participants had obvious psychological symptoms during the epidemic of COVID-19. The psychological symptoms of the college students were anxiety (61.64%), fear (58.39%), conformity (49.49%), invulnerability (26.11%), insensitivity (21.49%) and rebelliousness (12.41%). In addition, about 6.16% students had insomnia and 2.83% had the symptoms of in-appetite.

Moreover, the results of the survey also presented that psychological symptoms had no significant difference with regard to the gender, residence and annual household income while the financial level of the family had an obvious influence on insensitivity symptoms during the epidemic period. The survey also revealed that the senior students experienced more fear and anxiety than the freshmen due to the worry about the academic study delay and practice courses, graduation and employment.

Author Contributions: Conceptualization, J.H.; methodology, Y.L.; software, L.Q.; investigation, Y.S.; writing—original draft preparation, Y.L.; writing—review and editing, J.H. All authors have read and agreed to the published version of the manuscript.

Funding: This research was funded by Teaching Reform Research Project of Hubei Province, grant number 2018245. The APC was funded by Teaching Reform Research Project of Hubei Province.

Institutional Review Board Statement: The study was conducted according to the guidelines of the Declaration of Helsinki and approved by Ethics Committee of Wuhan University of Science and Technology (protocol code 20200407, 4 February 2021).

Informed Consent Statement: Informed consent was obtained from all subjects involved in the study.

Data Availability Statement: The data presented in this study are available on request from the corresponding author.

Conflicts of Interest: The authors declare no conflict of interest.

References

1. Hu, B.; Guo, H.; Zhou, P.; Shi, Z.-L. Characteristics of SARS-CoV-2 and COVID-19. *Nat. Rev. Microbiol.* **2021**, *19*, 141–154. [CrossRef] [PubMed]
2. Xue, D.; Liu, T.; Chen, X.; Liu, X.; Chao, M. Data on media use and mental health during the outbreak of COVID-19 in China. *Data Brief* **2021**, *35*, 106765. [CrossRef]
3. Sun, Z.; Zhang, H.; Yang, Y.; Wan, H.; Wang, Y. Impacts of geographic factors and population density on the COVID-19 spreading under the lockdown policies of China. *Sci. Total Environ.* **2020**, *746*, 141347. [CrossRef] [PubMed]
4. Olufadewa, I.I.; Adesina, M.A.; Ekpo, M.D.; Akinloye, S.J.; Iyanda, T.O.; Nwachukwu, P.; Kodzo, L.D. Lessons from the coronavirus disease 2019 (COVID-19) pandemic response in China, Italy, and the USA guide for Africa and low- and middle-income countries. *Glob. Health J.* **2021**. [CrossRef]
5. Wang, M.; Lu, S.; Shao, M.; Zeng, L.; Zheng, J.; Xie, F.; Lin, H.; Hu, K.; Lu, X. Impact of COVID-19 lockdown on ambient levels and sources of volatile organic compounds (VOCs) in Nanjing, China. *Sci. Total Environ.* **2021**, *757*, 143823. [CrossRef] [PubMed]
6. Tian, H.; Liu, Y.; Li, Y.; Wu, C.-H.; Chen, B.; Kraemer, M.U.G.; Li, B.; Cai, J.; Xu, B.; Yang, Q.; et al. An investigation of transmission control measures during the first 50 days of the COVID-19 epidemic in China. *Science* **2020**, *368*, 638–642. [CrossRef]
7. Tian, F.; Li, H.; Tian, S.; Yang, J.; Shao, J.; Tian, C. Psychological symptoms of ordinary Chinese citizens based on SCL-90 during the level I emergency response to COVID-19. *Psychiatry Res.* **2020**, *288*, 112992. [CrossRef] [PubMed]
8. Zhang, Q.; He, Y.-J.; Zhu, Y.-H.; Dai, M.-C.; Pan, M.-M.; Wu, J.-Q.; Zhang, X.; Gu, Y.-E.; Wang, F.-F.; Xu, X.-R.; et al. The evaluation of online course of Traditional Chinese Medicine for Medical Bachelor, Bachelor of Surgery international students during the COVID-19 epidemic period. *Integr. Med. Res.* **2020**, *9*, 100449. [CrossRef] [PubMed]
9. Song, M. Psychological stress responses to COVID-19 and adaptive strategies in China. *World Dev.* **2020**, *136*, 105107. [CrossRef]
10. Liu, S.; Yang, L.; Zhang, C.; Xiang, Y.-T.; Liu, Z.; Hu, S.; Zhang, B. Online mental health services in China during the COVID-19 outbreak. *Lancet Psychiatry* **2020**, *7*, e17–e18. [CrossRef]
11. Liu, Y.; Yue, S.; Hu, X.; Zhu, J.; Wu, Z.; Wang, J.; Wu, Y. Associations between feelings/behaviors during COVID-19 pandemic lockdown and depression/anxiety after lockdown in a sample of Chinese children and adolescents. *J. Affect. Disord.* **2021**, *284*, 98–103. [CrossRef]
12. Zhang, C.; Ye, M.; Fu, Y.; Yang, M.; Luo, F.; Yuan, J.; Tao, Q. The Psychological Impact of the COVID-19 Pandemic on Teenagers in China. *J. Adolesc. Health* **2020**, *67*, 747–755. [CrossRef]
13. Qiu, J.; Shen, B.; Zhao, M.; Wang, Z.; Xie, B.; Xu, Y. A nationwide survey of psychological distress among Chinese people in the COVID-19 epidemic: Implications and policy recommendations. *Gen. Psychiatry* **2020**, *33*. [CrossRef]
14. Wang, C.; Pan, R.; Wan, X.; Tan, Y.; Xu, L.; Ho, C.S.; Ho, R.C. Immediate Psychological Responses and Associated Factors during the Initial Stage of the 2019 Coronavirus Disease (COVID-19) Epidemic among the General Population in China. *Int. J. Environ. Res. Public Health* **2020**, *17*, 1729. [CrossRef] [PubMed]
15. Mazza, C.; Ricci, E.; Biondi, S.; Colasanti, M.; Ferracuti, S.; Napoli, C.; Roma, P. A Nationwide Survey of Psychological Distress among Italian People during the COVID-19 Pandemic: Immediate Psychological Responses and Associated Factors. *Int. J. Environ. Res. Public Health* **2020**, *17*, 3165. [CrossRef]
16. Copeland, W.E.; McGinnis, E.; Bai, Y.; Adams, Z.; Nardone, H.; Devadanam, V.; Rettew, J.; Hudziak, J.J. Impact of COVID-19 Pandemic on College Student Mental Health and Wellness. *J. Am. Acad. Child Adolesc. Psychiatry* **2021**, *60*, 134–141.e132. [CrossRef] [PubMed]
17. Chen, R.-n.; Liang, S.-w.; Peng, Y.; Li, X.-g.; Chen, J.-b.; Tang, S.-y.; Zhao, J.-b. Mental health status and change in living rhythms among college students in China during the COVID-19 pandemic: A large-scale survey. *J. Psychosom. Res.* **2020**, *137*, 110219. [CrossRef] [PubMed]
18. Davis, T.E.; Grills-Taquechel, A.E.; Ollendick, T.H. The Psychological Impact From Hurricane Katrina: Effects of Displacement and Trauma Exposure on University Students. *Behav. Ther.* **2010**, *41*, 340–349. [CrossRef]
19. Zhang, S.X.; Wang, Y.; Rauch, A.; Wei, F. Unprecedented disruption of lives and work: Health, distress and life satisfaction of working adults in China one month into the COVID-19 outbreak. *Psychiatry Res.* **2020**, *288*, 112958. [CrossRef]
20. Wang, C.; Pan, R.; Wan, X.; Tan, Y.; Xu, L.; McIntyre, R.S.; Choo, F.N.; Tran, B.; Ho, R.; Sharma, V.K.; et al. A longitudinal study on the mental health of general population during the COVID-19 epidemic in China. *Brain Behav. Immun.* **2020**, *87*, 40–48. [CrossRef]
21. Fu, W.; Yan, S.; Zong, Q.; Anderson-Luxford, D.; Song, X.; Lv, Z.; Lv, C. Mental health of college students during the COVID-19 epidemic in China. *J. Affect. Disord.* **2021**, *280*, 7–10. [CrossRef] [PubMed]
22. Jiang, R. Knowledge, attitudes and mental health of university students during the COVID-19 pandemic in China. *Child. Youth Serv. Rev.* **2020**, *119*, 105494. [CrossRef] [PubMed]
23. Schalet, B.D.; Cook, K.F.; Choi, S.W.; Cella, D. Establishing a common metric for self-reported anxiety: Linking the MASQ, PANAS, and GAD-7 to PROMIS Anxiety. *J. Anxiety Disord.* **2014**, *28*, 88–96. [CrossRef] [PubMed]
24. Ma, N.; Ma, H.; Li, L. Reading and analysis of the guiding principles of emergent psychological crisis intervention in the COVID-19. *Chin. J. Psychiatry* **2020**, *53*, 95–98.

25. Jones, N.M.; Thompson, R.R.; Dunkel Schetter, C.; Silver, R.C. Distress and rumor exposure on social media during a campus lockdown. *Proc. Natl. Acad. Sci. USA* **2017**, *114*, 11663–11668. [CrossRef]
26. Xie, X.; Zang, Z.; Ponzoa, J.M. The information impact of network media, the psychological reaction to the COVID-19 pandemic, and online knowledge acquisition: Evidence from Chinese college students. *J. Innov. Knowl.* **2020**, *5*, 297–305. [CrossRef]
27. Batra, K.; Sharma, M.; Batra, R.; Singh, T.P.; Schvaneveldt, N. Assessing the Psychological Impact of COVID-19 among College Students: An Evidence of 15 Countries. *Healthcare* **2021**, *9*, 222. [CrossRef]
28. Cao, W.; Fang, Z.; Hou, G.; Han, M.; Xu, X.; Dong, J.; Zheng, J. The psychological impact of the COVID-19 epidemic on college students in China. *Psychiatry Res.* **2020**, *287*, 112934. [CrossRef]
29. Cheung, T.; Wong, S.Y.; Wong, K.Y.; Law, L.Y.; Ng, K.; Tong, M.T.; Wong, K.Y.; Ng, M.Y.; Yip, P.S.F. Depression, Anxiety and Symptoms of Stress among Baccalaureate Nursing Students in Hong Kong: A Cross-Sectional Study. *Int. J. Environ. Res. Public Health* **2016**, *13*, 779. [CrossRef]
30. Li, Y.; Zhao, J.; Ma, Z.; McReynolds, L.S.; Lin, D.; Chen, Z.; Wang, T.; Wang, D.; Zhang, Y.; Zhang, J.; et al. Mental Health Among College Students During the COVID-19 Pandemic in China: A 2-Wave Longitudinal Survey. *J. Affect. Disord.* **2021**, *281*, 597–604. [CrossRef]
31. Budimir, S.; Pieh, C.; Dale, R.; Probst, T. Severe Mental Health Symptoms during COVID-19: A Comparison of the United Kingdom and Austria. *Healthcare* **2021**, *9*, 191. [CrossRef] [PubMed]
32. Moghanibashi-Mansourieh, A. Assessing the anxiety level of Iranian general population during COVID-19 outbreak. *Asian J. Psychiatry* **2020**, *51*, 102076. [CrossRef] [PubMed]
33. Shigemura, J.; Ursano, R.J.; Morganstein, J.C.; Kurosawa, M.; Benedek, D.M. Public responses to the novel 2019 coronavirus (2019-nCoV) in Japan: Mental health consequences and target populations. *Psychiatry Clin. Neurosci.* **2020**, *74*, 281–282. [CrossRef]
34. Rossell, S.L.; Neill, E.; Phillipou, A.; Tan, E.J.; Toh, W.L.; Van Rheenen, T.E.; Meyer, D. An overview of current mental health in the general population of Australia during the COVID-19 pandemic: Results from the COLLATE project. *Psychiatry Res.* **2021**, *296*, 113660. [CrossRef] [PubMed]
35. Chi, X.; Liang, K.; Chen, S.-T.; Huang, Q.; Huang, L.; Yu, Q.; Jiao, C.; Guo, T.; Stubbs, B.; Hossain, M.M.; et al. Mental health problems among Chinese adolescents during the COVID-19: The importance of nutrition and physical activity. *Int. J. Clin. Health Psychol.* **2020**, 100218. [CrossRef]
36. Hou, W.K.; Tong, H.; Liang, L.; Li, T.W.; Liu, H.; Ben-Ezra, M.; Goodwin, R.; Lee, T.M.-c. Probable anxiety and components of psychological resilience amid COVID-19: A population-based study. *J. Affect. Disord.* **2021**, *282*, 594–601. [CrossRef]

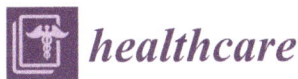

Article

Determinants of Behavioral Changes Since COVID-19 among Middle School Students

Jaewon Lee [1], Jennifer Allen [2], Hyejung Lim [3,*] and Gyuhyun Choi [4]

1. Department of Social Welfare, Inha University, Incheon 22212, Korea; j343@inha.ac.kr
2. School of Social Work, Michigan State University, East Lansing, MI 48823, USA; allenj66@msu.edu
3. School of Education, Korea University, Seoul 02841, Korea
4. Integrative Arts Therapy, Dongduk Women's University, Seoul 02748, Korea; toyou4048@uos.ac.kr
* Correspondence: nanapro@korea.ac.kr

Abstract: Middle school students are of particular interest when examining the impact of the COVID-19 pandemic because they are in a formative period for socioemotional development, and because they are not as mature as adults, making them more vulnerable to the effects of the current pandemic. This study seeks to examine determinants of protective behavior changes since COVID-19 among middle school students. Participants were recruited through an official online flatform used by public schools. The final sample included 328 middle school students in South Korea. A multiple linear regression was conducted to explore what factors influence protective behavior changes since COVID-19. Gender and health status were associated with protective behavior changes since COVID-19. Family satisfaction was positively associated with protective behavior changes. Levels of sanitation since COVID-19 and perceptions regarding the risk of COVID-19 were significantly related to protective behavior changes. This study suggests to consider three factors–individual, family, and environmental—in order to prevent middle school students from contracting and spreading the virus.

Keywords: COVID-19; protective behavior changes; individual; family; environmental factor

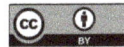

1. Introduction

As of mid-December 2020, the World Health Organization has reported nearly 74 million confirmed cases of COVID-19 and 1.6 million associated deaths worldwide [1]. In South Korea, there have been 48,570 confirmed cases and 659 associated deaths since COVID-19 emerged in Wuhan, China, in December 2019, and was identified as a new coronavirus in January 2020 [1,2]. By mid-February 2020, the number of cases in South Korea began to spread quickly, with the outbreak centered in the city of Daegu, southeast of Seoul [3]. The South Korean government implemented protective measures against the spread of COVID-19, including a national infectious disease plan stemming from the 2015 MERS outbreak; nationwide contact tracing efforts; and a ban on the export of face masks [4,5]. Such policies that encourage protective behaviors such as social distancing have been found to be effective in reducing the spread of COVID-19 [6]. Many of these social distancing measures, such as school closures and the subsequent transition to online learning, greatly affect adolescents, and researchers have found that the continued spread of COVID-19 has many deleterious effects on adolescents' mental, physical, and socioemotional health [7–13]. Therefore, it is of interest to examine the extent to which adolescents engage in protective behaviors against the spread of COVID-19, such as staying home and being more diligent about hygiene, and what determinants influence such behaviors, so that the spread of COVID-19 may be reduced [14].

1.1. Literature Review

1.1.1. Impacts of the COVID-19 Pandemic on Adolescents

Emerging research has shown that since the COVID-19 pandemic emerged, adolescents are at increased risk for various mental and physical health issues [7,10,11,13,15,16]. In a longitudinal study of adolescents in Shanghai, China conducted from January to March 2020, adolescents' physical activity decreased significantly, from an average of 540 min per week to 105 min per week [13]. In a 22-week longitudinal study of Australian adolescents, there was also a significant decrease in physical activity after the government of New South Wales implemented social distancing policies [17]. Similar findings were also reported in a sample of adolescents in southern Croatia, with physical activity levels particularly decreasing among boys [16].

Adolescents are also at increased risk for negative mental health outcomes since the beginning of the COVID-19 pandemic [10,11,15]. A review of the preliminary literature indicated an increased risk of posttraumatic stress disorder, depressive and anxiety symptoms among adolescents since the pandemic emerged [11]. Additionally, in a longitudinal study with Norwegian adolescents, the prevalence of mental distress increased significantly from February 2019 to June 2020 [15]. Moreover, in a survey of Canadian adolescents, stress related to the pandemic was associated with increased feelings of loneliness and depression [10].

1.1.2. Determinants of Adolescents' Protective Behavior Changes Since COVID-19

Utilizing Bronfenbrenner's ecological perspective on human development, determinants at multiple levels of the ecological system (e.g., individual and family) impact adolescents' protective behavior changes since COVID-19 [18]. Such protective changes may include increased handwashing; wearing a face mask; keeping distance from others; and working or attending school from home [14]. One determinant of protective behavior changes among adolescents that has emerged in the literature at the individual level is gender [16,19–23]. Compared to their female counterparts, male adolescents in Norway, Poland and Jordan, and young adult men in Switzerland were less likely to report protective handwashing behaviors [19–21,23]. Further, female adolescents in Poland and young adult women in Switzerland reported higher compliance with social distancing behaviors than their male counterparts, while no statistically significant difference by gender was found in a sample of adolescents in the United States [20–22]. Across studies, females were also found to be more likely than males to use hand sanitizer, avoid touching their face, and wear a face mask [19–21].

Another determinant of protective behaviors is one's perception of the risk of COVID-19 [24–27]. In an online survey of Chinese adolescents, results showed that perception of COVID-19 risk positively affected their understanding of and participation in social distancing behaviors [27]. Additionally, results of a survey of adults in Qatar found that the more highly they rated the danger of COVID-19, the more likely they were to socially distance [24]. Similarly, in a sample of adults in Hong Kong, a structural equation model revealed that perceptions of COVID-19 risk significantly affected compliance with protective measures (e.g., handwashing, social distancing) [25]. Further, researchers administered a survey to adults in Portugal and found that anxiety regarding COVID-19 and fear of death from COVID-19 significantly predicted protective behaviors, mediated by one's perception of their own perceived risk [26].

Moreover, at the family level, the main determinant that has been examined in the context of protective behavioral changes since COVID-19 is low parental monitoring [21]. Among Swiss young adults, low parental monitoring was associated with lower COVID-19 protective behavior compliance [21]. However, family factors such as conflict and emotion expression were related with COVID-19 stressors [28]. Thus, it is of interest to determine how COVID-19 stressors affect such family factors, which thereby may influence protective behaviors against COVID-19 with the intention to reduce the spread of COVID-19 and associated stressors.

1.1.3. The Current Study

The unprecedented, rapid spread of COVID-19 has negatively affected mankind. Middle school students are of particular interest when examining the impact of the COVID-19 pandemic because they are in a formative period for socioemotional development, and because they are not as mature as adults, making them more vulnerable to the effects of the current pandemic. Although middle school students are greatly affected by COVID-19, there are few studies looking at how COVID-19 affects them. In particular, we do not know how their behaviors and lives have changed since COVID-19. Thus, this study explores the relationships between possible indicators and protective behavior changes among middle school students since the COVID-19 pandemic began. This study seeks to (1) examine how individual factors such as age, gender and physical health influenced protective behavior changes since COVID-19; (2) investigate how family factors such as closeness and communication quality influenced protective behavior changes; and (3) explore how environmental factors such as levels of sanitation since COVID-19 and perceptions regarding the risk of COVID-19 influenced protective behavior changes since the beginning of the COVID-19 pandemic.

2. Methods

2.1. Participants and Sampling

Participants were recruited through an official online flatform used by public schools. The flatform is used as a communication tool between the schools and students and all students are able to receive notices from the school through the flatform. For this study, the target population was limited to middle school students enrolled in a public school in Gyeonggi province, the most populous area in South Korea. Participants were a convenience sample of middle school students. Data was collected from September to October 2020. Questionnaires were created in Google Forms and a link for the online survey was distributed through the public school's online flatform. To protect students' rights and improve the quality of the items, the questionnaires were evaluated and refined by experts, such as a middle school teacher. Participants received a $2 gift card as an incentive, and it took about twenty minutes to complete the survey. A total of three hundred fifteen four students participated. We excluded participants who declined consent to participate, either by themselves or by their caregivers. 26 respondents did not consent to participate so we excluded them in the final sample. As a result, the final sample included three-hundred twenty-eight participants. Even though this study does not contain any private identifiable information, this study was approved by the Institutional Review Board (#200810-1A). Further, given that the participants are not adults, a consent form was provided to both middle school students and their caregivers. Only middle school students whose caregivers also agreed with the participation engaged in this study. In addition, we did not collect any private information such as name, address, etc.

2.2. Measures

2.2.1. Protective Behavior Changes Since COVID-19

This scale measured to what extent middle school students changed their behaviors since the emergence of the COVID-19 pandemic. Participants were asked if they had/were "decreased outdoor activities", "reduced frequency of social gatherings", "more careful about cleanliness", and "increased time at home". This measurement consisted of four items which were rated on a five-point Likert-type scale. Response options for all items ranged from 1 (strongly disagree) to 5 (strongly agree). All responses were summed with higher scores indicating greater behavioral changes since COVID-19. Cronbach's α of behavioral changes since COVID-19 was 0.70 in this study ($M = 16.85$; $SD = 2.82$; ranging from 4 to 20).

2.2.2. Individual Factors

Age and gender were included as determinants in this study. In addition, respondents reported on their health status, which was measured via the Health Status subscale [29,30]. This measure consists of five items which are rated on a five-point Likert-type scale. Middle school students responded to the following questions: "I am in good physical health", "My body is in good physical shape", "I am a well-exercised person", "My body needs a lot of work in be in excellent physical shape", and "My physical health is in need of attention." The response options were as follows: Not at all characteristic of me; slightly characteristic of me; somewhat characteristic of me; moderately characteristic of me; and very characteristic of me. Two items were reverse-coded before analysis. We summed all items and higher scores indicated that respondents had greater physical health status. In this study, this scale had a Cronbach's alpha of 0.67 ($M = 16.23$; $SD = 3.63$; ranging from 6 to 25).

2.2.3. Family Factors
Family Satisfaction

The Family Satisfaction Scale was used to measure how satisfied respondents were with their family members [31]. This scale consists of ten items with a five-point Likert-type scale. For each item, participants were asked to indicate whether they were very dissatisfied, somewhat dissatisfied, generally satisfied, very satisfied, or extremely satisfied. Specific statements include the following: "The degree of closeness between family members", "Your family's ability to cope with stress", "The quality of communication between family members", and "Your family's ability to resolve conflicts." Each item was summed with higher scores indicating greater levels of family satisfaction. The Family Satisfaction Scale items in this study had a Cronbach's alpha of 0.92 ($M = 38.77$; $SD = 7.50$; ranging from 12 to 50).

Subjective Poverty

Respondents reported levels of subjective poverty by answering "In your circumstances, do you consider your household's economic status to be good or bad?" This question was derived from the Leyden Poverty Line [32]. The response options were as follows: very bad, bad, insufficient, sufficient, good, and very good. In this study, those who answered very bad, bad, or insufficient were regarded as being in poverty, while those who reported sufficient, good, or very good were considered as not being in poverty.

2.2.4. Environmental Factors
Levels of Sanitation Since COVID-19

Middle school students indicated to what extent they had changed their daily sanitation activities since COVID-19. They were queried whether they "Wash hands frequently", "Avoid touching own face", "Do not share personal items", or are "reluctant to go to crowded places due to hygiene problems." The respondents indicated their levels of sanitation since COVID-19 by choosing one of the following: strongly disagree, disagree, neutral, agree, or strongly agree. Each item was summed, with higher scores indicating greater levels of sanitation since COVID-19. The Cronbach's α of the five-point Likert-type scale was 0.71 ($M = 16.42$; $SD = 2.72$; ranging from 8 to 20).

Perceptions Regarding the Risk of COVID-19

Respondents stated to what extent they were aware of COVID-19. This scale consisted of four items which were rated on a five-point Likert-type scale with response options ranging from 1 (strongly disagree) to 5 (strongly agree). The specific items were as follows: COVID-19 is different than flu; [I] do not know when COVID-19 is gone, [COVID-19] damage[s] my health status, and [COVID-19] negatively influence[s] my daily life (e.g., by decreased frequency of dining out). The items were summed and higher scores indicated greater perception of risk regarding COVID-19. Cronbach's α of this scale was 0.70 ($M = 18.06$; $SD = 2.23$; ranging from 10 to 20).

2.3. Analysis Strategy

Analysis of variance and chi-squared tests were used to examine gender differences in individual, family, and environmental factors. A multiple linear regression was conducted to explore what factors influence protective behavior changes since COVID-19. Statistical Package for the Social Sciences (SPSS) 22.0 (IBM, Armonk, NY, USA) was employed to investigate the relationships between indicators and protective behavior changes since COVID-19. In the multiple linear regression model, individual factors were first considered, and then family factors and environmental factors sequentially addressed in the model. In other words, individual factors were included in model 1 while family factors were entered in model 2 with individual factors. Environmental factors were lastly added in model 3. Figure 1 shows the research design for the current study.

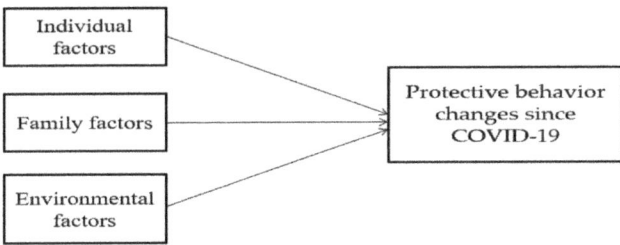

Figure 1. Research Design.

3. Results

Table 1 shows the descriptive statistics of variables used in the current study and gender differences in the dependent variable. There is a difference in protective behavior changes since COVID-19 between middle school boys and girls. Middle school girls had greater behavioral changes (17.20) than middle school boys (16.40) since the COVID-19 pandemic. Girls showed more decreased outdoor activities compared to boys (4.19 vs. 3.94), more reduced frequency of social gatherings (4.34 vs. 4.03), and more increased time at home (4.68 vs. 4.49). The average age of the middle school students was 14.4 years old. Slightly more than one-fourth of the total sample reported that they subjectively perceived being in poverty. The average scores for health status, family satisfaction, levels of sanitation since COVID-19, and perceptions regarding the risk of COVID-19 were 16.23, 38.77, 16.42, and 18.06, respectively.

Table 2 indicates which factors significantly influenced protective behavior changes since COVID-19 among middle school students. Model 1 includes individual factors and reveals that gender was associated with protective behavior changes since COVID-19 ($\beta = 0.77$, $p < 0.05$). When family factors were entered into model 2, girls were still more likely to have greater protective behavior changes since COVID-19 as compared to boys ($\beta = 0.76$, $p < 0.05$). Health status was negatively related to protective behavior changes since COVID-19 ($\beta = -0.12$, $p < 0.01$). Regarding family factors, family satisfaction was positively associated with protective behavior changes ($\beta = 0.12$, $p < 0.001$). Once COVID-19 environmental factors were included in model 3, gender, health status, and family satisfaction remained significant ($\beta = 0.68$, $p < 0.05$; $\beta = -0.14$, $p < 0.001$; $\beta = 0.06$, $p < 0.01$). For COVID-19 environmental factors, both levels of sanitation since COVID-19 and perceptions regarding the risk of COVID-19 were significantly related to protective behavior changes since COVID-19 ($\beta = 0.27$, $p < 0.001$; $\beta = 0.35$, $p < 0.001$).

Table 1. Descriptive Statistics for Variables Included in the Study.

Variable	Boys ($n = 146$) % or Mean (SD)	Girls ($n = 182$) % or Mean (SD)	Total ($n = 328$)	p
Protective behavior changes since COVID-19	16.40 (3.25)	17.20 (2.38)	16.85 (2.82)	*
Individual factors				
Age	14.41 (.74)	14.37 (1.19)	14.39 (1.01)	
Health status	16.52 (3.76)	15.99 (3.53)	16.23 (3.63)	
Family factors				
Subjective poverty	28.1%	27.5%	27.7%	
Family satisfaction	38.95 (7.14)	38.63 (7.80)	38.77 (7.50)	
Environmental factors				
Levels of sanitation since COVID-19	16.51 (2.94)	16.35 (2.52)	16.42 (2.72)	
Perceptions regarding the risk of COVID-19	17.90 (2.30)	18.19 (2.18)	18.06 (2.23)	

Note: * $p < 0.05$; Significant difference between males and females.

Table 2. Regression Results of Unstandardized Coefficients (standard error), Predicting Protective Behavior Changes Since COVID-19.

Variables	Protective Behavior Changes Since COVID-19					
	Model 1		Model 2		Model 3	
(Constant)	17.05 (2.38)		15.03 (2.30)		4.66 (2.46)	
Individual factors						
Gender (girl)	0.77 (0.31)	*	0.76 (0.30)	*	0.68 (0.27)	*
Age	0.01 (0.15)		0.07 (0.15)		0.06 (0.14)	
Health status	−0.05 (.04)		−0.12 (0.04)	**	−0.14 (0.04)	***
Family factors						
Subjective poverty			−0.30 (0.34)		−0.30 (0.31)	
Family satisfaction			0.12 (0.02)	***	0.06 (0.02)	**
Environmental factors						
Levels of sanitation since COVID-19					0.27 (0.06)	***
Perceptions regarding the risk of COVID-19					0.35 (0.06)	***

Note. * $p < 0.05$. ** $p < 0.01$. *** $p < 0.001$.

4. Discussion

The principal purpose of the current study was to examine determinants of protective behavior changes since COVID-19 in the context of three dimensions: individual, family, and environmental. This study revealed how individual, family, and environmental determinants influenced protective behavior changes among middle school students in South Korea since the emergence of the COVID-19 pandemic. Even though all people, regardless of their demographics or socioeconomic status, have been greatly influenced by the unprecedented spread of COVID-19, middle school students are at particular risk because of the importance of the adolescent years for development [33]. Given that little is known about protective behavior changes since COVID-19 among middle school students, the present study contributes to understanding the determinants of COVID-19 protective behavior changes in this population. This study indicated that both individual and family factors were important to understand protective behavior changes. Further, levels of sanitation since COVID-19 and perception of risk regarding COVID-19 also influenced protective behavior changes among middle school students.

Individual factors that influenced protective behavior changes since COVID-19 among middle school students included gender and perceived health status. This study indicated that there is a gender difference in the protective behavior changes since the coronavirus outbreak. Middle school girls showed that they were more inactive since COVID-19 compared to middle school boys. More specifically, girls reported decreased outdoor activities, reduced frequency of social gatherings, and increased time at home. Generally, being inactive may be perceived in a negative way, but the meaning during the coronavirus pandemic could be understood to be more careful and cautious so as not to be infected by the virus. In general, adolescent boys are more likely than adolescent girls to engage in risky behaviors [34], which in the time of COVID-19, may manifest as engaging in social activities. Greater behavior changes during the coronavirus pandemic means that people are less likely to be infected, indicating that middle school boys should be educated to be more careful to avoid the spread of COVID-19. That greater health status was related to fewer protective behavior changes since COVID-19 demonstrated that healthy individuals may underestimate the risks of coronavirus and therefore continue to behave as they did before the pandemic. That is, healthy people may think that they are able to overcome the virus even if they are infected and think that the coronavirus is similar to the seasonal flu. However, given higher death rates around the world due to the virus and the unprecedented influence on the global economy and individuals' lives [35], everyone should be very careful not to be infected, regardless of health status. Seemingly healthy people are not immune from coronavirus infections and negative consequences, but even if they have a mild infection, they can be a vector for transmitting the virus to the most vulnerable, such as older adults or those with underlying conditions that make them more at risk. Thus, even healthy middle school students must participate in preventive measures, such as social distancing, in order to protect themselves and other people.

This study confirmed that some family factors were also related to protective behavior changes since coronavirus emerged. Households' economic resources were not related to such behavioral changes, while family satisfaction was associated with the behavioral changes. The specific protective behavior changes include reduced outdoor time with friends and increased time at home due to social distancing. If people have negative family situations, spending more time together at home due to COVID-19-related policies may lead to conflict and other negative outcomes [36]. On the other hand, middle school students who have good relationships with their family members may be more accepting of spending more time at home. That is, individuals with higher family satisfaction may be more likely to engage in such COVID-19 preventive practices by staying home with their family members, leading them to be more protected from coronavirus disease. However, middle school students who have more conflicts and disharmony with parents or siblings may be exposed to higher risks of COVID-19 through behaviors which may expose them to the virus. That is, improved relationships between children and parents or siblings can result in protective behavior changes related to social distancing, leading to decreased risks of coronavirus infection among middle school students.

It is also important to pay attention to environmental factors related to COVID-19 to understand protective behavior changes since the coronavirus disease emerged. This study revealed that higher levels of sanitation since COVID-19 and greater perception of risk related to COVID-19 results in greater protective behavior changes among middle school students. In other words, environmental changes due to the virus have an impact on middle school students' behaviors. Middle school students who increase their sanitation behaviors may also be more likely to follow social distancing guidelines and therefore be at decreased risk for coronavirus infection. Thus, it is critical for middle school students to be educated about the importance of sanitary behaviors during the COVID-19 pandemic. This education on sanitary behaviors can be helpful to prevent the spread of coronavirus as middle school students change their behaviors to protect themselves from COVID-19. We recommend that this education includes the following: the importance of frequent hand washing; not touching one's face; not sharing personal items; and avoiding going to crowded places. In addition, middle school students who better perceived the risks of COVID-19 showed greater changes in their daily behaviors, thereby lowering their potential exposure to coronavirus. As middle school students are still maturing and spend most of their time at home and school, the role of parents and teachers is important to increase their perceptions regarding the risk of COVID-19. That is, adults who are responsible for the health of middle school children should first understand the risks of COVID-19, because they are a primary source to teach the children about the risks of COVID-19 [23].

However, along with receiving information from parents and other adults, children are likely to access and retrieve information from social media such as Instagram, Facebook, Twitter, etc. [19]. Given that social media provides both true and false information [37], it is imperative to teach middle school children how to distinguish correct information about COVID-19 from inaccurate information.

5. Conclusions

This study indicated the importance of environmental factors to influence behaviors that decrease the risk of COVID-19 infection. After a year, the COVID-19 pandemic is still affecting people around the world; however, little is known about determinants of protective behavior changes among middle school students since COVID-19, which helps middle school students be at lower risk of being infected by COVID-19. This study contributes to literature related to COVID-19, particularly among middle school students, and suggests to consider three factors–individual, family, and environmental—in order to prevent middle school students from contracting and spreading the virus.

Even though this study sheds light middle school students' protective behavior changes since the beginning of the COVID-19 pandemic, findings should be interpreted in the context of limitations. First, this study was conducted in South Korea, so behavioral changes among middle school students in other countries might be different from those in South Korea. Thus, cultural differences should be considered if the findings are to be applied to other settings. Second, additional factors can influence protective behavior changes since COVID-19, and we recommend that extra variables should be included in future studies. Third, this study focuses on middle school students regardless of disability status. Children with disabilities may have different determinants of protective behavior changes since the COVID-19 to consider. Therefore, we suggest that future studies focus on children with disabilities to identify if they differ from children without disabilities in terms of factors influencing protective behavior changes since the COVID-19 pandemic. Fourth, we calculated the sample size using a sample size calculator [38] with 5.24 confidence interval and 95% confidence level. The sample size needed in this study was 349; however, we recommend that an advanced power analysis or sample size estimation should be considered in future studies. Fifth, this survey needed to be completed during September and October 2020. Due to limited time and budget, we chose a convenience sample.

Author Contributions: Conceptualization, J.L., and H.L.; Data curation, H.L.; Formal analysis, H.L.; Investigation, J.L.; Methodology, J.L.; Project administration, H.L., and G.C.; Resources, G.C.; Writing—original draft, J.L., and J.A.; Writing—review and editing, J.A. All authors have read and agreed to the published version of the manuscript.

Funding: This research received no external funding.

Institutional Review Board Statement: The study was conducted according to the guidelines of the Declaration of Helsinki, and approved by the Institutional Review Board of Inha University (#200810-1A).

Informed Consent Statement: Informed consent was obtained from all subjects involved in the study.

Data Availability Statement: The data presented in this study are available on request from the corresponding author. The data are not publicly available due to ethical reasons.

Conflicts of Interest: The authors declare no conflict of interest.

References

1. World Health Organization. WHO Coronavirus Disease (COVID-19) Dashboard. 2020. Available online: https://covid19.who.int/ (accessed on 19 December 2020).
2. Keni, R.; Alexander, A.; Nayak, P.G.; Mudgal, J.; Nandakumar, K. COVID-19: Emergence, spread, possible treatments, and global burden. *Front. Public Health* **2020**, *8*, 216. [CrossRef] [PubMed]
3. Shim, E.; Tariq, A.; Choi, W.; Lee, Y.; Chowell, G. Transmission potential and severity of COVID-19 in South Korea. *Int. J. Infect. Dis.* **2020**, *93*, 339–344. [CrossRef] [PubMed]

4. Kim, J.-H.; An, J.A.-R.; Min, P.; Bitton, A.; Gawande, A.A. How South Korea responded to the Covid-19 outbreak in Daegu. *NEJM Catal. Innov. Care Deliv.* **2020**, *1*. [CrossRef]
5. You, J. Lessons from South Korea's Covid-19 policy response. *Am. Rev. Public Adm.* **2020**, *50*. [CrossRef]
6. McGrail, D.J.; Dai, J.; McAndrews, K.M.; Kalluri, R. Enacting national social distancing policies corresponds with dramatic reduction in COVID19 infection rates. *PLoS ONE* **2020**, *15*, e0236619. [CrossRef]
7. Bates, L.C.; Zieff, G.; Stanford, K.; Moore, J.B.; Kerr, Z.Y.; Hanson, E.D.; Gibbs, B.B.; Kline, C.E.; Stoner, L. COVID-19 impact on behaviors across the 24-hour day in children and adolescents: Physical activity, sedentary behavior, and sleep. *Children* **2020**, *7*, 138. [CrossRef]
8. Dall, C. South Korea among Several Nations Eyeing Lockdowns. Available online: https://www.cidrap.umn.edu/news-perspective/2020/12/south-korea-among-several-nations-eyeing-lockdowns (accessed on 19 December 2020).
9. Dighe, A.; Cattarino, L.; Cuomo-Dannenberg, G.; Skarp, J.; Imai, N.; Bhatia, S.; Gaythorpe, K.A.M.; Ainslie, K.E.C.; Baguelin, M.; Bhatt, S.; et al. Response to COVID-19 in South Korea and implications for lifting stringent interventions. *BMC Med.* **2020**, *18*, 1–12. [CrossRef]
10. Ellis, W.E.; Dumas, T.M.; Forbes, L.M. Physically isolated by socially connected: Psychological adjustment and stress among adolescents during the initial COVID-19 crisis. *Can. J. Behav. Sci.* **2020**, *52*, 177–187. [CrossRef]
11. Guessoum, S.B.; Lachal, J.; Radjack, R.; Carretier, E.; Minassian, S.; Benoit, L.; Moro, M. Adolescent psychiatric disorders during the COVID-19 pandemic and lockdown. *Psychiatry Res.* **2020**, *291*. [CrossRef]
12. Torales, J.; O'Higgins, M.; Castadelli-Maia, J.M.; Ventriglio, A. The outbreak of COVID-19 coronavirus and its impact on global mental health. *Int. J. Soc. Psychiatry* **2020**, *66*, 317–320. [CrossRef] [PubMed]
13. Xiang, M.; Zhang, Z.; Kuwahara, K. Impact of COVID-19 pandemic on children and adolescents' lifestyle behavior larger than expected. *Prog. Cardiovasc. Dis.* **2020**, *63*, 531–532. [CrossRef] [PubMed]
14. Vannabouathong, C.; Devji, T.; Ekhtiari, S.; Chang, Y.; Phillips, S.A.; Zhu, M.; Chagla, Z.; Main, C.; Bhandari, M. Novel coronavirus COVID-19: Current evidence and evolving strategies. *J. Bone Jt. Surg. Am.* **2020**, *102*, 734–744. [CrossRef] [PubMed]
15. Hafstad, G.S.; Sætren, S.S.; Wentzel-Larsen, T.; Augusti, E.-M. Longitudinal change in adolescent mental health during the COVID-19 outbreak: A prospective population-based study of teenagers in Norway. *Lancet* **2020**. [CrossRef]
16. Sekulic, D.; Blazevic, M.; Gilic, B.; Kvesic, I.; Zenic, N. Prospective analysis of levels and correlates of physical activity during COVID-19 pandemic and imposed rules of social distancing: Gender specific study among adolescents from southern Croatia. *Sustainability* **2020**, *12*, 4072. [CrossRef]
17. Munasinghe, S.; Sperandei, S.; Freebairn, L.; Conroy, E.; Jani, H.; Marjanovic, S.; Page, A. The impact of physical distancing policies during the COVID-19 pandemic on health and well-being among Australian adolescents. *J. Adolesc. Health* **2020**, *67*, 653–661. [CrossRef]
18. Bronfenbrenner, U. *The Ecology of Human Development: Experiments by Nature and Design*; Harvard University Press: Cambridge, MA, USA, 1979.
19. Dardas, L.A.; Khalaf, I.; Nabolsi, M.; Nassar, O.; Hulasa, S. Developing an understanding of adolescents' knowledge, attitudes, and practices toward COVID-19. *J. Sch. Nurs.* **2020**, *36*, 430–441. [CrossRef]
20. Guzek, D.; Skolmowska, D.; Glabska, D. Analysis of gender-dependent personal protective behaviors in a national sample: Polish adolescents' COVID-19 experience (PLACE-19) study. *Int. J. Environ. Res. Public Health* **2020**, *17*, 5770. [CrossRef]
21. Nivette, A.; Ribeaud, D.; Murray, A.; Steinhoff, A.; Bechtiger, L.; Hepp, U.; Shanahan, L.; Eisner, M. Non-compliance with COVID-19-related public health measures among young adults in Switzerland: Insights from a longitudinal cohort study. *Soc. Sci. Med.* **2021**, *268*. [CrossRef]
22. Oosterhoff, B.; Palmer, C.A.; Wilson, J.; Shook, N. Adolescents' motivations to engage in social distancing during the COVID-19 pandemic: Associations with mental and social health. *J. Adolesc. Health* **2020**, *67*, 179–185. [CrossRef]
23. Riiser, K.; Helseth, S.; Haraldstad, K.; Torbjornsen, A.; Richardsen, K.R. Adolescents' health literacy, health protective measures, and health-related quality of life during the Covid-19 pandemic. *PLoS ONE* **2020**, *15*, e0238161. [CrossRef]
24. Abdelrahman, M. Personality traits, risk perception, and protective behaviors of Arab residents in Qatar during the COVID-19 pandemic. *Int. J. Ment. Health Addict.* **2020**. [CrossRef] [PubMed]
25. Chong, Y.Y.; Chien, W.T.; Cheng, H.Y.; Chow, K.M.; Kassianos, A.P.; Karekla, M.; Gloster, A. The role of illness perceptions, coping, and self-efficacy on adherence to precautionary measures for COVID-19. *Int. J. Environ. Res. Public Health* **2020**, *17*, 6540. [CrossRef] [PubMed]
26. Paison, R.; Paiva, T.O.; Fernandes, C.; Barbosa, F. The AGE effect on protective behaviors during the COVID-19 outbreak: Sociodemographic, perceptions and psychological accounts. *Front. Psychol.* **2020**, *11*, 2785. [CrossRef]
27. Xie, K.; Liang, B.; Dulebenets, M.A.; Mei, Y. The impact of risk perception on social distancing during the COVID-19 pandemic in China. *Int. J. Environ. Res. Public Health* **2020**, *17*, 6256. [CrossRef]
28. Westrupp, E.; Bennett, C.; Berkowitz, T.; Youssef, G.; Toumbourou, J.; Tucker, R.; Andrews, F.; Evans, S.; Teague, S.; Karantzas, G.; et al. Child, parent, and family mental health and functioning in Australia during COVID-19: Comparison to pre-pandemic data. *PsyArXiv* **2020**. [CrossRef]
29. Snell, W.E.; Johnson, G.; Lloyd, P.J.; Hoover, W. The development and validation of the Health Orientation Scale: A measure of psychological tendencies associated with health. *Eur. J. Personal.* **1991**, *5*, 169–183. [CrossRef]

30. Snell, W.E.; Johnson, G.; Lloyd, P.J.; Hoover, W. The Health Orientation Scale (HOS). Available online: https://www.midss.org/content/health-orientation-scale-hos (accessed on 20 December 2020).
31. Olson, D.H. FACES IV and the Circumplex Model: Validation study. *J. Marital Fam. Ther.* **2011**, *37*, 64–80. [CrossRef]
32. Kapteyn, A.; Kooreman, P.; Willemse, R. Some methodological issues in the implementation of subjective poverty definitions. *J. Hum. Resour.* **1988**, *23*, 222–242. [CrossRef]
33. Viner, R.M.; Ross, D.; Hardy, R.; Kuh, D.; Power, C.; Johnson, A.; Wellings, K.; McCambridge, J.; Cole, T.J.; Kelly, Y.; et al. Life course epidemiology: Recognising the importance of adolescence. *J. Epidemiol. Community Health* **2015**, *69*, 719–720. [CrossRef]
34. Auerbach, R.P.; Tsai, B.; Abela, J.R.Z. Temporal relationships among depressive symptoms, risky behavior engagement, perceived control, and gender in a sample of adolescents. *J. Res. Adolesc.* **2010**, *20*. [CrossRef]
35. Nicola, M.; Alsafi, Z.; Sohrabi, C.; Kerwan, A.; Al-Jabir, A.; Iosifidis, C.; Agha, M.; Agha, R. The socio-economid implications of the coronavirus pandemic (COVID-19): A review. *Int. J. Surg.* **2020**, *78*, 185–193. [CrossRef] [PubMed]
36. Pereda, N.; Diaz-Faes, D.A. Family violence against children in the wake of COVID-19 pandemic: A review of current perspectives and risk factors. *Child Adolesc. Psychiatry Ment. Health* **2020**, *14*. [CrossRef] [PubMed]
37. Meel, P.; Vishwakarma, D.K. Fake news, rumor, information pollution in social media and web: A contemporary survey of state-of-the-arts, challenges and opportunities. *Expert Syst. Appl.* **2020**, *153*. [CrossRef]
38. Creative Research Systems. Sample Size Calculator. 2021. Available online: https://covid19.who.int/ (accessed on 3 January 2021).

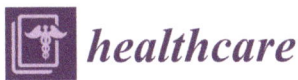

Article

Perceptions and Preventive Practices Regarding COVID-19 Pandemic Outbreak and Oral Health Care Perceptions during the Lockdown: A Cross-Sectional Survey from Saudi Arabia

Abdullah Alassaf, Basim Almulhim, Sara Ayid Alghamdi and Sreekanth Kumar Mallineni *

Department of Preventive Dental Science, College of Dentistry, Majmaah University,
Al-Majmaah 11952, Saudi Arabia; am.assaf@mu.edu.sa (A.A.); b.almulhim@mu.edu.sa (B.A.);
Sa.mohammed@mu.edu.sa (S.A.A.)
* Correspondence: s.mallineni@mu.edu.sa; Tel.: +966-507780161

Citation: Alassaf, A.; Almulhim, B.; Alghamdi, S.A.; Mallineni, S.K. Perceptions and Preventive Practices Regarding COVID-19 Pandemic Outbreak and Oral Health Care Perceptions during the Lockdown: A Cross-Sectional Survey from Saudi Arabia. *Healthcare* **2021**, *9*, 959. https://doi.org/10.3390/healthcare9080959

Academic Editors: Manoj Sharma and Kavita Batra

Received: 11 July 2021
Accepted: 22 July 2021
Published: 29 July 2021

Publisher's Note: MDPI stays neutral with regard to jurisdictional claims in published maps and institutional affiliations.

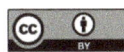

Copyright: © 2021 by the authors. Licensee MDPI, Basel, Switzerland. This article is an open access article distributed under the terms and conditions of the Creative Commons Attribution (CC BY) license (https://creativecommons.org/licenses/by/4.0/).

Abstract: Aims: The study aimed to evaluate perceptions and preventive practices regarding the COVID-19 pandemic and oral health care perceptions during the lockdown in the Saudi Arabian population. Materials and Method: This cross-sectional study was performed by collecting the data from individuals belonging to various parts of the Saudi Arabian Population through an online self-reported questionnaire. The questionnaire had two main parts: first comprised of demographic data include the region of residence, gender, nationality, age, the number of family members, monthly income of the family, and the second was further divided into three sections of perception (P), practice (PRA) and oral health care practice (D) questions. All these (P, PRA, and D) were analyzed by comparing all of the demographic characteristics. Statistical analysis was performed using SPSS IBM (version 21.0), and statistical significance was set at a 5% level. Results: Overall, 2013 participants (54% males and 46% females) contributed to the Saudi Arabia study. Only 5% of non-Saudis live in Saudi Arabia were participated in the study, while the majority of participants were of 21–40 years age group (45%), 59% of having more than five family members, and 60% of them had ≤10 K Suadi riyal monthly income respectively. The majority of the participants were from Riyadh (33.7%) and Asir (25.1%) in the study. Overall, 89.5% of the participants were aware of the COVID-19 global pandemic. The majority of the participants (55%) from Saudi Arabia utilized the Ministry of Health website, a source of information regarding COVID-19. However, 56.5% of the participants had COVID-19 related perception, and 74.3% followed an appropriate preventive practice. Approximately 60% had good oral health practice. The study participants showed mixed opinions on perceptions regarding COVID-19, preventive practice, and oral health practices. Conclusion: The present study suggested that the Saudi Arabian population has good attention to COVID-19, but preventive practice and oral health perception need better awareness to control this novel virus spread. The Ministry of Health website utilized as a significant source of information among the Saudi Arabian population regarding COVID-19.

Keywords: Coronavirus; Saudi Arabia; perception; COVID-19; prevention

1. Introduction

Coronavirus disease is referred to as "COVID-19" and is caused by a novel respiratory virus [1] and this single-stranded RNA virus belongs to a Coronaviridae family [2,3]. It was transmitted initially from animal-to-human and then human-to-human [1,4]. The governments and public health organizations have adopted numerous measures worldwide to improve awareness, raise knowledge, and increase preventive practice to control COVID-19 transmission [5,6]. It originated from China at the end of the year 2019 and subsequently circulated globally [7]. The first positive case reported of COVID-19 was by the Ministry of Health (MOH), Kingdom of Saudi Arabia, on 2nd March 2020. Eventually, the number of positive cases was accelerated in a month, and it has become a big challenge for healthcare professionals [7]. As of 31 December 2020, 362,714 cases were registered in Saudi Arabia [8]. The government authorities of Saudi Arabia have focused on precautionary measures with general population interest [9]. These include lockdown, airport and border surveillance, quarantine of suspicious and infected patients, and infection control training for healthcare workers [10]. In addition, public places are at potential risk of spreading COVID-19 to family and friends, and colleagues [11]. Therefore, it became essential that the public know the disease and preventive practices suggested by health authorities. COVID-19 transmits through air droplets, contaminated surfaces, mucus membranes and secretions from the nose or mouth, or eyes, and close contact with infected persons [12,13]. COVID-19 cases are usually symptomatic; however, recently, asymptomatic patients have also been reported, which has become a significant concern for health care professionals. Dry cough, fatigue, fever, dyspnea, and myalgia, commonly reported symptoms in COVID-19 positive individuals. Subsequently, an Italian study reported that there will be an alteration in smell and taste in individuals with COVID-19 [14]. Additional observed symptoms include abdominal pain, headache, diarrhea, and sore throat. The severe stage of COVID-19 is characterized by septic shock, acute respiratory distress syndrome, bleeding, coagulation disorders, and metabolic acidosis [15,16].

The world health organization (WHO) recommends specific preventive personal hygiene measures, including using face masks, repeated handwashing with water and soap, using hand sanitizers, avoiding touching mouth, eyes, and nose frequently, cleanliness, and social distancing well as careful handling of purchased products. These measures are very strictly acclaimed to control the spread of COVID-19 disease and to protect the people from this pandemic. Nevertheless, a lack of understanding of the COVID-19 risk factors among people has been observed worldwide [10,17]. People's understanding and adherence to preventive measures play an essential part in controlling the contraction of COVID-19 [9]. Di Lorenzo and Di Trolio [16] opined that strict obedience to the rules proposed by health authorities might be useful in avoiding the transmission of COVID-19. This tractability depends on their awareness, perception, and preventive practice factors. Hence, there is a need for a survey to check for the perception, preventive practice, and oral health care perceptions in Saudi Arabia. Oral health care professionals are at potential risk of acquiring COVID-19 because most dental procedures are aerosol generated [5,13,18]. It also impacted the people whether to seek dental treatment during this COVID-19 pandemic or not. Nonetheless, there is no data available on the oral health care perceptions of the Saudi Arabian population. However, lack of awareness and inadequate understanding of the people at risk has led to the COVID-19 pandemic outbreak of this disease, resulting in colossal morbidity and mortality worldwide. Henceforth, the study was aimed to evaluate perceptions and preventive practices regarding the COVID-19 pandemic and oral health care perceptions during the lockdown: a population-based cross-sectional survey from Saudi Arabia.

2. Materials and Method

The Ethical Committee Clearance was obtained from Majmaah University, Al-Majmaah, Saudi Arabia, under IRB No: MUREC-June-10/Com-2020/32-3. This cross-sectional survey was conducted from 1 June 2020 to 31 July 2020 among the people from Saudi Arabia, and the self-administered questionnaire was sent through digital platforms online via google forms. The questionnaire comprised two main parts: first part consisted of demographic data including the region of residence (Riyadh, Al Baha, Makkah, Qassim, Northern Border region, Tabuk, Jazan, Asir, Hail, Madinah, Najran, Eastern, and Al Jouf), gender (male and female), nationality (Saudi and Non-Saudi), age in years ($\leq$20, 21–40, 41–60, >60), number of family members ($\leq$5 and >5), and monthly income of the family ($\leq$10 KSAR and >10 K Saudi riyal (SAR). The second part had three sections as follows: Six questions for perception (P), preventive practice (PRA), and three questions for oral health care perception (D), shown in Table 1. A pilot survey was conducted among the team members that filled and reviewed all the questions. The changes were made accordingly prior to the distribution of the questionnaire among the participants. The responses obtained from the pilot study were not included in the final data analysis. The validation of the questionnaire was completed and translated into Arabic by a native speaker (AA) and edited prior to distribution. The translations were made accessible in English and Arabic languages. The participants made it an easy and understandable form. The effect of age, gender, nationality, number of family members, and monthly income was considered for evaluating P, PRA, and D regarding COVID-19. The questionnaire was sent as a link via social media to the Saudi Arabian population using Google form. The recruitment and consent to participate in the study followed the participants' willingness to complete the questionnaire. In the perception of the feasibility of analysis "yes" as a positive response and "no" as a negative response. Similarly, we followed the same criteria for all the domains. The mean percentages of the positive responses for all the questions were used for the measurement. The Chi-square tests were used for comparisons of percentages. All the demographic characteristics of participants were presented using summary statistics. The statistical analysis was performed using IBM SPSS Statistics (Version 21.0. Armonk, NY, USA: IBM Corp); statistical significance was set at a 5% level.

Table 1. Questions related to perception (P), preventive practice (PRA), and oral health care perceptions (D).

No.	Questions
P1	Do you think the Corona virus incidence can be reduced by staying at home and not meeting with others during lockdown?
P2	Do you know the symptoms of the Coronavirus?
P3	Do you think your monthly income is going to effect during this lockdown period?
P4	Do you monitor the daily new cases of affected people by Coronavirus in your city during the lockdown period?
P5	Do you recommend your family members and neighbors use face masks and gloves for safety when they go out during this lockdown period?
P6	How do you think the financial consumption rate will be affected during this lockdown period?
PRA1	If symptoms of Coronavirus exist, would you disclose and go to the hospital for screening?
PRA2	Do you feel an embarrassment in others' non-shaking hands because of the customs and traditions during this COVID-19 lockdown period?
PRA3	Are you using a face mask and washing hands with soap and water or sanitizer to prevent Coronavirus transmission in lockdown period?
PRA4	To what extent do you commit to lockdown period and curfew laws?
PRA5	Are you able to refuse your family visitors during the COVID-19 lockdown period?
PRA6	Are you maintaining social distance?
D1	Have you felt any dental pain or discomfort during this COVID-19 period?
D2	Do you prefer to visit the dentist personally during this COVID-19 period?
D3	Are you happy to make a call with a dentist explaining your dental problems rather than visiting the dentist personally before treatment?

3. Results

A total of 2013 participants responded in the study from various regions of Saudi Arabia (Figure 1). The majority of the participants were from the Riyadh region (33.7%), followed by the Asir region (21.5%). Amongst the participants' males were 1088 (54%), and 925 (46%) were females. The distribution of study participants was shown in Figure 1.

The majority (95%) of the total participants was Saudis by nationality, and 59% of the participants confirmed that they had more than five members in their family, and 60% had a monthly income of less than 10 K. The age-wise distribution of participants was ≤20 years (17%), 21–40 years (46%), 41–60 years (34%), and >60 years (3%), respectively. All the demographic characteristics were summarized in Figure 2. The Saudi Arabian population utilized various sources for information on COVID-19, that include the MOH website, Saudi Arabia (55%), social media (24%), news channels (16%), and WHO (4%) see Figure 3.

The mean percentage of positive answers of perception, preventive practices, and oral health practices percentage of achieved scores were summarized in Table 2 based on the study population's demographic characteristics. Amongst the participants' females (70%), Saudis (69%), 41–60 years age group (66%), ≤5 family members (71%), and ≤10 K SAR salary (70%) showed higher mean percentages for perceptions on COVID-19. For preventive practices, females (78%), Saudis (75%), 41–60 years age group (70%), >5 family members (75%), and >10 K SAR salary (75%) achieved a higher mean percentage. While females (26%), Saudis (32%), 41–60 years age group (35%), ≤5 family members (50%), and ≤10 K SAR salary (33%) mean percentages achieved for oral health care perception among population live in Saudi Arabia (Table 2).

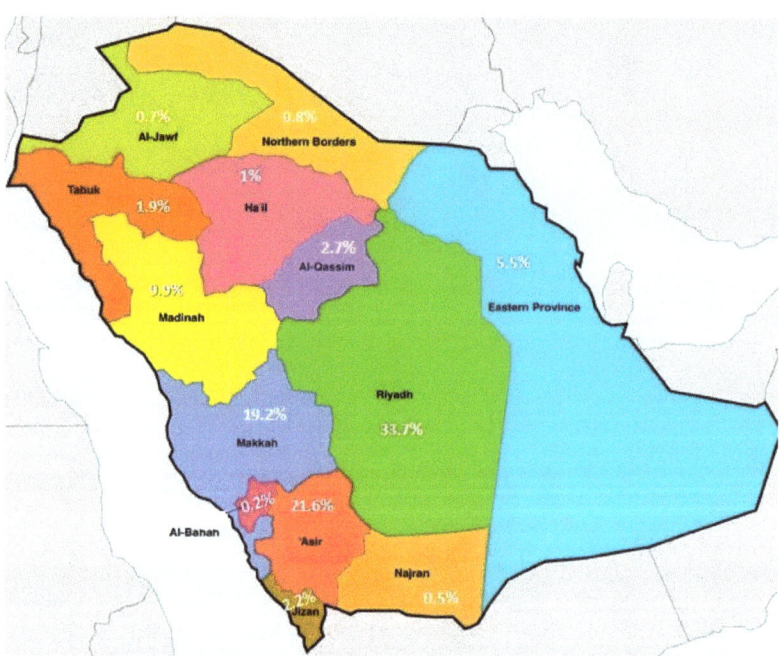

Figure 1. Distribution of participants based on the region in Saudi Arabia.

Table 2. Overall mean percentage scores of perception, preventive practice, and oral health care perceptions.

Parameters		Perception (P)	Preventive Practice (PRA)	Oral Health Care Perception (D)
Gender	Female	70%	78%	26%
	Male	67%	71%	21%
Nationality	Non Saudi	68%	72%	29%
	Saudi	69%	75%	32%
Age	<20 year	59%	67%	35%
	21–40	65%	67%	31%
	41–60	66%	70%	31%
	>60 year	65%	67%	26%
Family member	1–5	71%	74%	50%
	>5	67%	75%	48%
Income	<	70%	74%	33%
	>	68%	75%	31%

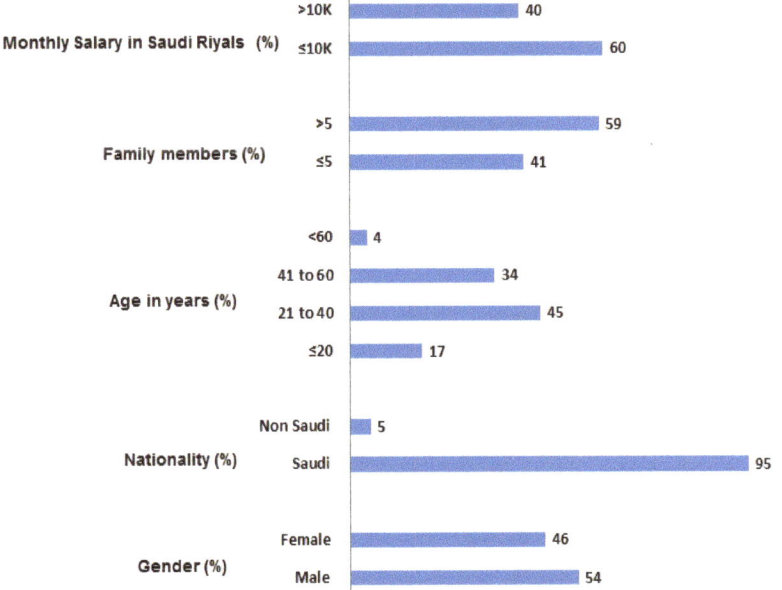

Figure 2. Demographic data of population participated in the study.

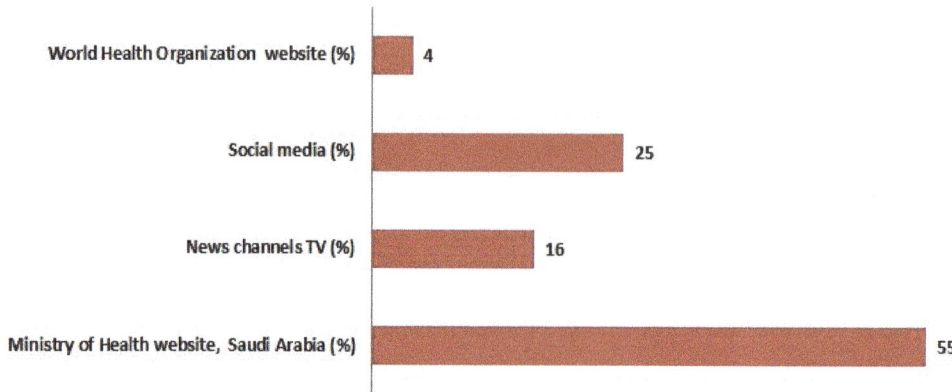

Figure 3. Details of the source of information utilized by the Saudi Arabian population participated in the study.

The present study results showed that approximately 89.5% of the participants had proper awareness about COVID-19 and its symptoms (Table 3). Understanding the COVID-19 symptoms was significantly less among the non-Saudi participants than the Saudi participants ($p = 0.000$). Awareness on COVID-19 was found to be more in females, those below 60 years of age, having less than five family members, and monthly income of more than 10 K ($p > 0.05$). Amongst the participants' females (90%), Saudis (90%), 41–60 years age group (91%), ≤5 family members (91%), and >10 K SAR salary (91%). There was a statistically significant difference evident in the comparison of nationality and monthly salary. The majority of the males (35%), non-Saudis (55%), and participants belongs to 21–40 years age group (39%), and ≤ 10 SAR monthly salary opined that monthly income is going to affect in lockdown period and the statistically significant was evident ($p > 0.05$). Regarding the financial consumption rate during the lockdown, 55% of the females and 54% of ≤ 10 K SAR monthly salary participants stated that the financial consumption rate would affect ($p < 0.05$). The nationality, various age groups, and the family members' number showed no statistical difference ($p > 0.05$).

The majority of the participants were willing to disclose to hospital authorities if they have suspicious symptoms of COVID-19. Amongst them are males (95%), Saudis (94%), 41–60 years age group (96%), ≤5 family members (95%), and >10 K SAR salary (95%) willing to disclose to the hospital authorities. All the comparisons showed statistically significant ($p < 0.05$). Mixed views were observed regarding preventive practices (wearing a facemask, social distancing, washing hands with soap, and using sanitizer) among the Saudi Arabian population during pandemic based on gender, nationality, age groups, number of family members, and monthly income (Table 4). On the other hand, regarding following the curfew rules, females (69%) than males (54%), Saudis (61%) than non-Saudis (57%), age group belongs to more than 60% (71%) than other age groups committed to the restrictions. There was a statistical difference evident among these comparisons ($p > 0.05$). Regarding refusing family visitors during the lockdown period, two-thirds of females and participants belong to the 41–60 years age group ($p < 0.05$). Regarding the study participants' oral health perceptions, overall, significantly fewer people experienced dental pain or dental discomfort during the lockdown period (Table 5). Amongst, the majority of them were females (37%), non-Saudis (30%), <20 years (38%), and ≤10 K SAR (32%), the findings were statistically significant ($p < 0.05$). Significantly a smaller number of the participants were willing to visit the dentist during the lockdown period, which includes 17% of males ($p > 0.05$), 16% of Saudis ($p < 0.05$), 19% of ≤20 years age group ($p > 0.05$), 35% of them having more than five family members ($p < 0.05$) and 19% ≤ 10 K SAR ($p < 0.05$).

Table 3. Comparison of the effect of demographic factors on perception score during covid-19 in Arabian population.

Questions	Gender			Demographic Factor Nationality			Age (in years)					Family Members			Income (SAR)		
	F	M	p Value	NS	S	p Value	<20	21-40	41-60	>60	p Value	<5	>5	p Value	<10 K	>10 K	p Value
P1	93%	90%	0.03 *	82%	92%	<0.001 *	92%	90%	93%	87%	0.20	93%	90%	0.05	90%	92%	0.09
P2	90%	89%	0.80	87%	90%	0.03 *	87%	89%	91%	85%	0.29	91%	88%	0.11	87%	91%	<0.001 *
P3	31%	35%	<0.001 *	55%	32%	<0.001 *	21%	39%	32%	34%	<0.001 *	34%	34%	0.08	41%	29%	<0.001 *
P4	60%	63%	0.05	52%	62%	<0.001 *	44.%	64%	66%	69%	<0.001 *	65%	59%	0.01 *	58%	64%	<0.001 *
P5	90%	79%	<0.001 *	83%	84%	<0.001 *	85%	84%	85%	81%	0.14	86%	83%	0.14	87%	82%	<0.001 *
P6	55%	48%	0.01 *	46%	52%	0.79	27%	26%	29%	36%	0.13	54%	50%	0.08	54%	50%	0.04 *

Perception Questions—P1, P2, P3 and P4; F = Female; M = Male; NS = None Saudi; S = Saudi; SAR = Saudi riyal; * Significant $p < 0.05$.

Table 4. Comparison of effect of demographic factors on preventive practice score during COVID-19 in Arabian population.

Questions	Gender			Demographic Factor Nationality			Age (years)					Family Members			Income (SAR)		
	F	M	p Value	NS	S	p Value	<20	21-40	41-60	>60	p Value	<5	>5	p Value	<10 K	>10 K	p Value
PRA1	92%	95%	<0.001 *	88%	94%	<0.001 *	89%	93%	96%	91%	<0.001 *	95%	93%	0.01 *	90%	95%	<0.001 *
PRA2	66%	54%	<0.001 *	64%	59%	0.10	20%	27%	19%	10%	<0.001 *	58%	61%	0.48	58%	60%	0.68
PRA3	93%	89%	0.01	84%	91%	0.02 *	92%	92%	90%	83%	<0.001 *	92%	90%	0.16	92%	90%	0.41
PRA4	69%	54%	<0.001 *	57%	61%	<0.001 *	63%	58%	63%	71%	<0.001 *	58%	63%	0.44	62%	60%	0.31
PRA5	65%	60%	0.01	60%	63%	0.78	60%	58%	69%	67%	<0.001 *	63%	62%	0.52	61%	63%	0.13
PRA6	83%	75%	<0.001 *	77%	79%	0.04 *	79%	76%	82%	81%	0.18	78%	80%	0.39	79%	79%	0.21

Preventive practice Questions—P1, P2, P3 and P4; F = Female; M = Male; NS = None Saudi; S = Saudi; SAR = Saudi riyal; * Significant $p < 0.05$.

Table 5. Comparison of the effect of demographic factors on oral health care perception score.

| Questions | Demographic Factors ||||||||||||||||
| | Gender ||| Nationality ||| Age (in Years) |||||| Family Members ||| Income (SAR) |||
	F	M	p Value	NS	S	p Value	<20	21-40	41-60	>60	p Value	<5	>5	p Value	<10 K	>10 K	p Value
D1	37%	19%	<0.001 *	30%	27%	0.62	38%	28%	21%	9%	<0.001 *	27%	27%	0.11	32%	24%	<0.001 *
D2	15%	17%	0.37	9%	16%	<0.001 *	19%	18%	13%	13%	0.07	14%	18%	0.01 *	19%	14%	<0.001 *
D3	52%	52%	0.98	47%	53%	0.40	49%	48%	58%	56%	<0.001 *	53%	52%	0.01 *	49%	54%	<0.001 *

Oral health care perception questions—D1, D2, and D3 F = Female; M = Male; NS = None Saudi; S = Saudi; SAR = Saudi riyal; * Significant $p < 0.05$.

4. Discussion

Perceptions, preventive practices, and oral health practices among the Saudi Arabian population regarding the COVID-19 pandemic were assessed in the present study. This study is the first to discuss all these aspects among the Arabian population residing in various Saudi Arabia regions to the best of the authors' knowledge. In the present study, the overall awareness of COVID-19 was 89.5% of the study population. A similar observation was observed in the Cameroon population [19] found a similar score (84.19%). Contrarily, our findings did not agree with the African-based population study [3], where the authors found 73.5% of awareness regarding COVID-19 in their study population. Earlier, a similar survey in Saudi Arabian population was published in which the knowledge score was found to be 81.64%, which is less than the present study suggesting that the people of Saudi Arabian have a better understanding of the present scenario and are updating them with the COVID-19 knowledge [20]. Overall, 90% of the participants discerned that the incidence of COVID-19 could be minimized by staying at home and not meeting with others in public places during the lockdown period. This knowledge was significantly more in females than in males ($p = 0.000$). In addition, 89% of them knew about the symptoms of COVID-19. In a similar study by Honarvar et al. [21] in the Iranian population, it was found that only 4.8% of the participants were not aware of the symptoms of COVID-19, which suggests that the people of Saudi Arabia are more knowledgeable about the current global pandemic.

The overall perception in the present study was found to be 56.5%. A similar bi-national survey from the African population [3] observed 64% regarding COVID-19 among the study population. Thirty-six percent of the present study participants thought their monthly income would be affected during the lockdown period, and 61% monitor the daily new cases of affected people by COVID-19 in their city. Eighty-four percent recommend their family members and neighbors to use face masks and gloves for safety when they go out during the lockdown period, and 50% thought that the financial consumption rate would be decreased during the lockdown period. In the present study, perceptions were found more in females ($p = 0.000$), non-Saudi participants ($p = 0.000$), those below 60 years of age, those with more than five family members, and those having an income of less than 10 K ($p = 0.002$).

The overall preventive practice score in the present study was 74.3%. A practice score of 60.8% was observed in a similar study by Ngwewondo et al. [19] in the Cameroon population. In the present study, 93% of the participants agreed that if Coronavirus symptoms exist, they would disclose it and go to the hospital for screening ($p = 0.000$); 61% accepted that they feel an embarrassment in non-shaking hands with others because of the customs and traditions during this COVID-19 lockdown period, whereas 21.8% did not feel any embarrassment in non-shaking hands, in which females were significantly more in number than males ($p \leq 0.001$). In addition, 89.5% use a face mask and wash 1 s with soap and water or sanitizer to prevent Coronavirus transmission ($p \leq 0.001$). Sixty-one percent of the participants rated their commitment as 5, suggesting a total commitment to lockdown periods and curfew laws. 62.6% refused their family visitors during the COVID-19 lockdown period, and 79% maintained social distance ($p \leq 0.001$).

The overall oral health care perceptions were 60% in the present study. 74% of the participants did not experience any dental pain or discomfort during this COVID-19 period, whereas 26% had felt dental pain or discomfort during this COVID-19 period. 67.4% did not prefer to visit the dentist personally during this COVID-19 period, and 52% would like to call the dentist explaining their dental problems rather than visiting the dentist personally before treatment. In the present study, females were found to be more knowledgeable than males. Also, perception, preventive practice, and oral health care perception were more in females than males. Hence, more knowledge was associated with increased perception, more preventive practice, and oral health care perception in females in the present study. Honarvar et al. [21] studied the perception of COVID-19 among the Iranian population and found increased knowledge and preventive practice in females. Similar observations were made by Al-Hanawi et al. [20], Brug et al. [22], Bish and Michie [23]. In contrast, Ngwewondo et al. [19] have observed more preventive practice in males than females. Saudi participants were more knowledgeable than the non-Saudi participants in the present study ($p > 0.05$); nonetheless, perceptions were less among the Saudi participants than the non-Saudi participants. However, preventive practice and oral health care perception were more in Saudi participants than in the non-Saudi participants ($p < 0.05$). Hence, their increased knowledge was associated with higher preventive practice and oral health care perception. The perception was more in participants below 60 years of age. However, preventive practice and oral health care perception were found more in elderly participants over 60 years because older people are more prone to infectious diseases. The present study also observed more preventive practices in older people, and these findings are consistent with a Chinese study [18] and a Nigerian study [24] Zhang et al. [18]. This outcome explains that older people with or without comorbid diseases gained more preventive practices than other age groups. Similarly, increased age associated with an increased preventive approach was observed by Zhong et al. [18], Al-Hanawi et al. [20], and Lorfa et al. [24] in their respective studies. Honarvar et al. [22] have observed less knowledge and less preventive practice in the elderly age groups. Participants with less than five members were found to have more knowledge and oral health care perception, but the perception and preventive practice were found more in those with more than five family members. These differences were not statistically significant. None of the reported studies have reported family members' effect on perception and preventive practices regarding COVID-19 and oral health care perceptions during COVID-19. Perceptions, preventive practice, and oral health care perception were observed more in participants with a monthly income of more than 10 K, whereas perception was observed more in those with less than 10 K income ($p = 0.000$). Al-Hanawi et al. [20] have also found more awareness of COVID-19 in participants with higher income in their study.

The COVID-19 pandemic outbreak severely impacted the healthcare profession, especially in dentistry [6,8]. This pandemic has changed dental care providers' opinions and opinions of dental care receivers [25–27]. Almost 50% of participants from an American study reported delaying their dental appointments due to the COVID-19 pandemic [28]. Only a few participants preferred to visit the dental operatory. Comparing the gender, nationality, monthly income, and the number of family members showed statistical significance. However, no prior study compared these factors on dental visit preference during COVID-19 lockdown from Saudi Arabia. Comparatively, most survey participants preferred to have a telephonic conversation with the dentist before a dental appointment. The health authority provides guidelines for safe and effective dental practice during this pandemic outbreak [29]. The use of personal protection equipment (PPE), including N95 respirators, face shields, eye protection, surgical masks, and protective clothing, is strictly recommended to avoid the contraction of COVID-19 in the dental operatory. It explains the need for a telemedicine model in such pandemic situations. A recent article by Benzian and Niederman [26] explained SAFER dentistry that could benefit both the patients and dental care providers. Focusing on the source of information regarding COVID-19 amongst the people is also plays an essential role in perception and preventive practices. In the present study, only 4% of the participants relied on the WHO website. In Alanazei et al. [30] study, 18% of the participants preferred the WHO website. However, Alanazei et al. [20] findings are not comparable because they used multiple options for the source of information utilized for COVID-19. It has also been reported that the different sources of information had copious associations with the assurance in managing with concern to COVID-19 [31]. Participants in the present study used a multiplicity of sources for information concerning the COVID-19. The Saudi Arabia Ministry of Health website was utilized by most participants (55%) in the study to know information on COVID-19. Alanezi et al. [30] also reported similar findings. The authors reported that 65% of the participants utilized the Ministry of Health, Saudi Arabia, as a source of information. Furthermore, it explains the health authorities from Saudi Arabia were very successful in reaching people in the country with information regarding COVID-19 based on our study. Risk perceptions refer to people's spontaneous estimations of vulnerabilities they might be exposed to, with unwanted effects that the population associates with a precise cause [14,32,33]. Risk perception of a country means interpretations of the populations. Sharma et al. [34] used a fourth-generation multi-theory model (MTM) to explain and explore the hand-washing behavior among American college students.

A survey from Saudi Arabia also confirmed the risk perceptions regarding COVID-19 among dental undergraduate students [35]. A multinational study from 15 countries [36] reported that there need to develop a proper public health intervention to address college students' emotional and psychosocial needs during this COVID-19 Pandemic. A recent study [37] reported that dental specialists showed adequate knowledge regarding preventive measures. Furthermore, a recent study [38] suggested that it is imperative to promote the infection control protocols among dental students through training programs to avoid the potential risk of COVID-19. Cori et al. [39] opined that government authorities' administration of risk communication is required to establish consciousness and rationality. A recent study [40] found a higher prevalence rate of anxiety, depression, sleep problems, stress, and psychological distress among the general population during this pandemic outbreak. However, in the present study, we have not evaluated the psychological aspects of the populations. There is a need to evaluate the stress levels among the general population in Saudi Arabia. Based on the present study findings, the authors opine that the perception of risk regarding COVID-19 might associate with perceptions about COVID-19 and that will impact preventive behavior.

Limitations

A diversity of variables could predict the general population's reactions to the COVID-19 pandemic to avoid infection. The present study aimed to establish Saudi Arabian residents' perceptions, preventive practices regarding CVOID-19, and oral health practices during COVID-19. The present study utilized a limited number (2013) of participants from Saudi Arabian from various provinces, and studies with a larger sample size are recommended. The population from illiterate and unprivileged groups did not participate in the study. Therefore, the findings from these segments of the society were not gathered in the present study. A total of 2013 people participated from various Saudi Arabia regions, and the majority were from the Riyadh region (33.7%), followed by the Asir region (21.5%). The region-based analysis was not done in the present study. There was a comparatively remarkable difference among participants from the various areas. However, this could also be a limitation of the study. To the best of our knowledge, the present study qualifies as the first reported study from Saudi Arabia to the best of our knowledge assessed the perception, preventive practices, and oral health practices among the population in Saudi Arabia with concern to COVID-19. Other limitations include study design, self-administered questionnaire, convenience sampling, which cannot be generalized to the study findings. There was no equal distribution of the participants from various provinces of Saudi Arabia, and the majority of the study participants were from Riyadh and Asir. Nonetheless, the findings in the present study possibly will be used as a reference to explore variance with sample size made up of a population without internet access.

5. Conclusions

The present study concludes that although the knowledge is sufficient amongst the Saudi Arabian population, there is a need to improve participants' perception, preventive practice, and oral health care perceptions to improve their active involvement in controlling the COVID-19 transmission. The Ministry of Health Saudi Arabia website is the most reliable source of information COVID-19. The present study suggests that the Ministry of Health in Saudi Arabia successfully created awareness, and mixed responses were observed on preventive practices among the Saudi Arabian population. Comprehensive details of COVID-19 perceptions, preventive practices, and oral health care practices among the Saudi Arabian population based on gender, nationality, age groups, family members, and monthly incomes were discussed in this study.

Author Contributions: A.A. and B.A.; developed the concept, S.A.A. and S.K.M.; written the first draft. All the authors involved in reviewing and editing the manuscript. All authors have read and agreed to the published version of the manuscript.

Funding: This research received no external funding.

Institutional Review Board Statement: The Ethical Committee Clearance was obtained from Majmaah University, Al-Majmaah, Saudi Arabia, under IRB No: MUREC-June-10/Com-2020/32-3.

Informed Consent Statement: Informed consent was obtained from all subjects involved in the study.

Data Availability Statement: The data that support the findings of this study are available from the corresponding authors upon reasonable request.

Acknowledgments: The authors would like to thank the Deanship of Scientific Research at Majmaah University for supporting this work under Project Number No. R-2021-172.

Conflicts of Interest: The authors declare no conflict of interest.

References

1. Lai, C.C.; Shih, T.P.; Ko, W.C.; Tang, H.J.; Hsueh, P.R. Severe acute respiratory syndrome coronavirus 2 (SARS-CoV-2) and coronavirus disease-2019 (COVID-19): The epidemic and the challenges. *Int. J. Antimicrob. Agents* **2020**, *55*, 105924. [CrossRef]
2. Du, W.; Han, S.; Li, Q.; Zhang, Z. Epidemic update of COVID-19 in Hubei Province compared with other regions in China. *Int. J. Infect. Dis.* **2020**, *95*, 321–325. [CrossRef]
3. Hager, E.; Odetokun, I.A.; Bolarinwa, O.; Zainab, A.; Okechukwu, O.; Al-Mustapha, A.I. Knowledge, attitude, and perceptions towards the 2019 Coronavirus Pandemic: A bi-national survey in Africa. *PLoS ONE* **2020**, *15*, e0236918. [CrossRef] [PubMed]
4. Chen, J. Pathogenicity and transmissibility of 2019-nCoV-A quick overview and comparison with other emerging viruses. *Microbes Infect.* **2020**, *22*, 69–71. [CrossRef] [PubMed]
5. Seneviratne, C.J.; Lau, M.W.J.; Goh, B.T. The role of dentists in COVID-19 is beyond dentistry: Voluntary medical engagements and future preparedness. *Front. Med.* **2020**, *7*, 566. [CrossRef] [PubMed]
6. Meng, L.; Hua, F.; Bian, Z. Coronavirus Disease 2019 (COVID-19): Emerging and Future Challenges for Dental and Oral Medicine. *J. Dent. Res.* **2020**, *99*, 481–487. [CrossRef]
7. V'kovski, P.; Kratzel, A.; Steiner, S.; Stalder, H.; Thiel, V. Coronavirus biology and replication: Implications for SARS-CoV-2. *Nat. Rev. Microbiol.* **2020**, *28*, 1–16. [CrossRef] [PubMed]
8. Ministry of Health. Public Health—Novel Coronavirus (COVID-19). Available online: https://www.moh.gov.sa/en/HealthAwareness/EducationalContent/PublicHealth/Pages/corona.aspx (accessed on 1 May 2021).
9. Algaissi, A.A.; Alharbi, N.K.; Hassanain, M.; Hashem, A.M. Preparedness and response to COVID-19 in Saudi Arabia: Building on MERS expe-rience. *J. Infect. Public Health* **2020**, *13*, 834–838. [CrossRef]
10. Buerhaus, P.I.; Auerbach, D.I.; Staiger, D.O. Older Clinicians and the Surge in Novel Coronavirus Disease 2019 (COVID-19). *JAMA* **2020**, *323*, 1777–1778. [CrossRef] [PubMed]
11. Asaad, A.; El Sokkary, R.; Alzamanan, M.; El Shafei, M. Knowledge and attitudes towards Middle East respiratory sydrome-coronavirus (MERS-CoV) among health care workers in south-western Saudi Arabia. *East. Mediterr. Health J.* **2020**, *26*, 435–442. [CrossRef]
12. Wiersinga, W.J.; Rhodes, A.; Cheng, A.C.; Peacock, S.J.; Prescott, H.C. Pathophysiology, transmission, diagnosis, and treatment of Coronavirus disease 2019 (COVID-19): A review. *JAMA* **2020**, *324*, 782–793. [CrossRef]
13. Mallineni, S.K.; Innes, N.P.; Raggio, D.P.; Araujo, M.P.; Robertson, M.D.; Jayaraman, J. Coronavirus disease (COVID-19): Characteristics in children and considerations for dentists providing their care. *Int. J. Paediatr. Dent.* **2020**, *30*, 245–250. [CrossRef]
14. Bianco, M.R.; Modica, D.M.; Drago, G.D.; Azzolina, A.; Mattina, G.; De Natale, M.; Rossi, G.; Amata, M.; Canzoneri, G.; Manganaro, G.; et al. Alteration of Smell and Taste in Asymptomatic and Symptomatic COVID-19 Patients in Sicily, Italy. *EarNose Throat J.* **2021**, *100*, 182S–185S. [CrossRef]
15. Briguglio, M.; Pregliasco, F.E.; Lombardi, G.; Perazzo, P.; Banfi, G. The malnutritional status of the host as a virulence factor for new Coronavirus SARS-CoV-2. *Front. Med.* **2020**, *7*, 146. [CrossRef]
16. Di Lorenzo, G.; Di Trolio, R. Coronavirus Disease (COVID-19) in Italy: Analysis of risk factors and proposed remedial measures. *Front. Med.* **2020**, *7*, 140. [CrossRef] [PubMed]
17. Aldhuwayhi, S.; Shaikh, S.A.; Mallineni, S.K.; Varadharaju, V.K.; Thakare, A.A.; Khan, A.R.A.; Ziauddin, M.; Manva, M.Z. Occupational stress and stress busters utilized among Saudi dental practitioners during the COVID-19 pandemic outbreak. *Disaster Med. Public Health Prep.* **2021**, 1–21. [CrossRef]

18. Zhong, B.-L.; Luo, W.; Li, H.-M.; Zhang, Q.-Q.; Liu, X.-G.; Li, W.-T.; Li, Y. Knowledge, attitudes, and practices towards COVID-19 among Chinese residents during the rapid rise period of the COVID-19 outbreak: A quick online cross-sectional survey. *Int. J. Biol. Sci.* **2020**, *16*, 1745–1752. [CrossRef] [PubMed]
19. Ngwewondo, A.; Nkengazong, L.; Ambe, L.A.; Ebogo, J.T.; Mba, F.M.; Goni, H.O.; Nyunaï, N.; Ngonde, M.C.; Oyono, J.-L.E. Knowledge, attitudes, practices of/towards COVID 19 preventive measures and symptoms: A cross-sectional study during the exponential rise of the outbreak in Cameroon. *PLoS Negl. Trop. Dis.* **2020**, *14*, e0008700. [CrossRef]
20. Al-Hanawi, M.; Angawi, K.; Alshareef, N.; Qattan, A.M.N.; Helmy, H.Z.; Abudawood, Y.; AlQurashi, M.; Kattan, W.; Kadasah, N.A.; Chirwa, G.C.; et al. Knowledge, Attitude and Practice Toward COVID-19 Among the Public in the Kingdom of Saudi Arabia: A Cross-Sectional Study. *Front. Public Health* **2020**, *8*, 217. [CrossRef] [PubMed]
21. Honarvar, B.; Lankarani, K.B.; Kharmandar, A.; Shaygani, F.; Zahedroozgar, M.; Haghighi, M.R.R.; Ghahramani, S.; Honarvar, H.; Daryabadi, M.M.; Salavati, Z.; et al. Knowledge, attitudes, risk perceptions, and practices of adults toward COVID-19: A population and field-based study from Iran. *Int. J. Public Health* **2020**, *65*, 731–739. [CrossRef]
22. Brug, J.; Aro, A.R.; Oenema, A.; De Zwart, O.; Richardus, J.H.; Bishop, G.D. SARS Risk Perception, Knowledge, Precautions, and Information Sources, the Netherlands. *Emerg. Infect. Dis.* **2004**, *10*, 1486–1489. [CrossRef]
23. Bish, A.; Michie, S. Demographic and attitudinal determinants of protective behaviours during a pandemic: A review. *Br. J. Health Psychol.* **2010**, *15*, 797–824. [CrossRef] [PubMed]
24. Lorfa, S.K.; Ottu, I.F.A.; Oguntayo, R.; Ayandele, O.; Kolawole, S.O.; Gandi, J.C.; Dangiwa, A.L.; Olapegba, P.O. COVID-19 knowledge, risk per-ception, and precautionary behavior among Nigerians: A moderated mediation approach. *Front. Psychol.* **2020**, *11*, 566773.
25. Widyarman, A.S.; Bachtiar, E.W.; Theodorea, C.F.; Rizal, M.I.; Roeslan, M.O.; Djamil, M.S.; Santosa, D.N.; Bachtiar, B.M. COVID-19 Awareness Among Dental Professionals in Indonesia. *Front. Med.* **2020**, *7*, 589759. [CrossRef]
26. Benzian, H.; Niederman, R. A Dental Response to the COVID-19 Pandemic—Safer Aerosol-Free Emergent (SAFER) Dentistry. *Front. Med.* **2020**, *7*, 520. [CrossRef]
27. Tay, J.R.H.; Ng, E.; Ong, M.M.A.; Sim, C.; Tan, K.; Seneviratne, C.J. A Risk-Based Approach to the COVID-19 Pandemic: The Experience in National Dental Centre Singapore. *Front. Med.* **2020**, *7*, 562728. [CrossRef]
28. Kranz, A.M.; Gahlon, G.; Dick, A.W.; Stein, B.D. Characteristics of US adults delaying dental care due to the COVID-19 pandemic. *JDR Clin. Trans. Res.* **2021**, *6*, 8–14. [PubMed]
29. Bhumireddy, J.; Mallineni, S.K.; Nuvvula, S. Challenges and possible solutions in dental practice during and post COVID-19. *Environ. Sci. Pollut. Res.* **2021**, *28*, 1275–1277. [CrossRef]
30. AlAnezi, F.; Aljahdali, A.; Alyousef, S.; Alrashed, H.; AlShaikh, W.; Mushcab, H.; Alanzi, T. Implications of Public Understanding of COVID-19 in Saudi Arabia for Fostering Effective Communication Through Awareness Framework. *Front. Public Health* **2020**, *8*, 494. [CrossRef]
31. Wang, P.W.; Lu, W.H.; Ko, N.Y.; Chen, Y.L.; Li, D.J.; Chang, Y.P.; Yen, C.F. COVID-19-related information sources and the relationship with confidence in people coping with COVID-19: Facebook survey study in Taiwan. *J. Med. Internet Res.* **2020**, *22*, e20021. [CrossRef]
32. World Health Organization. COVID-2019 Situation Report [Internet]. Available online: https://www.who.int/docs/default-source/coronaviruse/situation-reports/20200215-sitrep-26-covid-19.pdf?sfvrsn=a4cc6787_2 (accessed on 1 May 2021).
33. Kaushik, M.; Agarwal, D.; Gupta, A.K. Cross-sectional study on the role of public awareness in preventing the spread of COVID-19 outbreak in India. *Postgrad. Med. J.* **2020**, 1–5. [CrossRef]
34. Sharma, M.; Batra, K.; Davis, R.E.; Wilkerson, A.H. Explaining Handwashing Behavior in a Sample of College Students during COVID-19 Pandemic Using the Multi-Theory Model (MTM) of Health Behavior Change: A Single Institutional Cross-Sectional Survey. *Healcare* **2021**, *9*, 55. [CrossRef]
35. Almulhim, B.; Alassaf, A.; Alghamdi, S.; Alroomy, R.; Aldhuwayhi, S.; Aljabr, A.; Mallineni, S.K. Dentistry Amidst the COVID-19 Pandemic: Knowledge, Attitude, and Practices Among the Saudi Arabian Dental Students. *Front. Med.* **2021**, *8*, 654524. [CrossRef]
36. Batra, K.; Sharma, M.; Batra, R.; Singh, T.; Schvaneveldt, N. Assessing the Psychological Impact of COVID-19 among College Students: An Evidence of 15 Countries. *Healthcare* **2021**, *9*, 222. [CrossRef]
37. Aldhuwayhi, S.; Mallineni, S.K.; Sakhamuri, S.; Thakare, A.A.; Mallineni, S.; Sajja, R.; Sethi, M.; Nettam, V.; Mohammad, A.M. Covid-19 Knowledge and Perceptions Among Dental Specialists: A Cross-Sectional Online Questionnaire Survey. *Risk Manag. Health Policy* **2021**, *14*, 2851–2861. [CrossRef] [PubMed]
38. Batra, K.; Urankar, Y.; Batra, R.; Gomes, A.F.; Kaurani, P. Knowledge, Protective Behaviors and Risk Perception of COVID-19 among Dental Students in India: A Cross-Sectional Analysis. *Healthcare* **2021**, *9*, 574. [CrossRef] [PubMed]
39. Cori, L.; Bianchi, F.; Cadum, E.; Anthonj, C. Risk Perception and COVID-19. *Int. J. Environ. Res. Public Health* **2020**, *17*, 3114. [CrossRef]
40. Lakhan, R.; Agrawal, A.; Sharma, M. Prevalence of Depression, Anxiety, and Stress during COVID-19 Pandemic. *J. Neurosci. Rural. Pract.* **2020**, *11*, 519–525. [CrossRef]

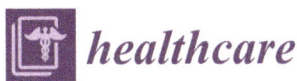

Article

Student Health Implications of School Closures during the COVID-19 Pandemic: New Evidence on the Association of e-Learning, Outdoor Exercise, and Myopia

Ji Liu [1], Baihuiyu Li [1], Qiaoyi Chen [2,*] and Jingxia Dang [3,*]

[1] Faculty of Education, Shaanxi Normal University, Xi'an 710062, China; jiliu@snnu.edu.cn (J.L.); lilyli000627@outlook.com (B.L.)
[2] School of Basic Medical Sciences, Xi'an Jiaotong University, Xi'an 710061, China
[3] The First Affiliated Hospital, Xi'an Jiaotong University, Xi'an 710061, China
* Correspondence: qychen203@xjtu.edu.cn (Q.C.); jxdang2000@126.com (J.D.)

Abstract: The coronavirus disease 2019 (COVID-19) pandemic forced many education systems to consider alternative remote e-learning modalities, which have consequential behavioral and health implications for youth. In particular, increased e-learning engagement with digital screens and reduction in outdoor activities are two likely channels posing adverse risks for myopia development. This study investigated the association between e-learning screen use, outdoor activity, lighting condition, and myopia development among school-age children in China, during the first wave of the COVID-19 pandemic. Data were collected from 3405 school-age children attending primary, lower-secondary, and upper-secondary schools in China. Univariate parametric and nonparametric tests, and multivariate logistic regression analysis were used. Findings show that each diopter hour increase in daily e-learning screen use is significantly associated with progression of myopia symptoms (OR: 1.074, 95% CI: 1.058–1.089; $p < 0.001$), whereas engaging in outdoor exercise four to six times per week (OR: 0.745, 95% CI: 0.568–0.977; $p = 0.034$) and one to three times per week (OR: 0.829, 95% CI: 0.686–0.991; $p = 0.048$) is associated with a lower likelihood of myopia progression than none at all. In addition, we found that indoor lighting that is either "too dim" (OR: 1.686, 95% CI: 1.226–2.319; $p = 0.001$) or "too bright" (OR: 1.529, 95% CI: 1.007–2.366; $p = 0.036$) is significantly associated higher likelihood of myopic symptoms. Findings in this study uncover the less observable vision consequences of the COVID-19 pandemic on youths through digital online learning and highlight the importance of considering appropriate mitigation strategies to deal with this emerging public health challenge.

Keywords: e-learning; youth and children health; visual health; myopia; COVID-19

1. Introduction

The outbreak and spread of the coronavirus disease 2019 (COVID-19) pandemic have greatly impacted education systems worldwide, with more than 190 countries/territories closing schools partially or in full during peak months, affecting at least 1.5 billion school-age children [1]. In order to minimize learning disruptions and to resume proper functioning of educational activities, more than 60 educational systems have elected to partially re-open schools by offering online remote instruction and supplementary digital learning modalities [2]. While replacing print textbooks with e-learning arrangements and swapping in-person classroom teaching with online video conferencing provides reasonable and timely solutions to deal with challenges of pandemic-led school closures, the adverse vision consequences associated with these ad hoc emergency and crisis arrangements may be substantial [3], especially considering new eye-use routines during the pandemic and its consequent behavioral implications for young children whose sensory function is going through critical development [4]. Notably, the current global increase in myopia, which is a major factor contributing to irreversible blindness, has become a leading public health concern. By 2050, it is projected that 50% of the world population will be affected [5], which underscores the need to investigate the relevant risk factors, as well as potential mitigation strategies to combat this public health challenge.

In this regard, it is hypothesized that the reduction of outdoor activity due to school closures and home confinement, coupled with the overlapping increase in e-learning digital screen use as a result of remote e-learning arrangements, presents critical vision development risk factors that could propel higher myopia incidence and progression by re-shaping daily physical and learning behaviors. On the one hand, intensive use of digital screens for extended periods of time can have detrimental effects on children's vision health development. Particularly, since eye development occurs throughout early stages of life, in vivo studies have suggested that prolonged near-vision stimulation can result in premature hyperopic defocus, which triggers compensating axial myopic eye growth and refractive vision development [6]. On the other hand, reduction in outdoor activities due to pandemic-led social-distancing measures and closure of public venues may present another less favorable environmental factor influencing young children's vision health. In this regard, prior research has found outdoor playtime was associated with better uncorrected visual acuity [7], especially because outdoor lighting is categorically less fluorescent than indoors [8].

Notwithstanding, the potential vision health risks propagated by new norms in instructional and learning arrangements amidst the ongoing COVID-19 pandemic will likely add to an already serious global youth vision crisis [9]. Importantly, early myopia (near-sightedness) onset and progression among young children are especially concerning, not only because of its widespread prevalence and difficulty in proper mitigation applications [10] but also due to critically associated risks of lasting vision impairment [11]. In particular, excessive axial elongation of the eye associated with early myopia increases later-life risks of vision disease complications including macular degeneration, posterior staphyloma, retinal detachment, cataract, and glaucoma that could lead to blindness [12]. More worryingly, myopia onset is becoming increasingly prevalent among young children, particularly for girls in higher grades and in urban areas [13–15]. Studies have also shown that the earlier children become myopic, the more likely they are to develop high myopia, and the worse the prognosis [16].

From a physiological perspective, in vivo studies employing infant monkeys have suggested that extended relative peripheral hyperopic defocus stimulation can alter central refractive development [17], which could likely induce compensating axial myopic eye growth and premature refractive vision development [18]. For instance, it has been shown using inflammatory markers in mice that blue light emitted from computer screens has potentially harmful effects on the retinal pigment epithelium, which may result in axial elongation and development of pathological myopia [19]. In addition, outdoor eye use under natural light is commonly associated with increased depth of focus and reduced eye strain, which are inversely related to axial elongation [20]. In studies employing in vivo models, visual experiments have shown that poor lighting conditions can lead to excessive vitreous chamber lengthening, such that low-light level can result in axial elongation and refractive myopic excursions, while high-light level is associated with lower rates of form-deprivation myopia [21].

Critically, while existing studies have independently examined near-vision electronic use, outdoor activity, and lighting condition, the interrelated relationship among the three have not been assessed in conjunction, and their relative risks are unknown. In this study, we examined the association between digital screen use, outdoor activity, lighting condition, and myopia development among school-age children in China during the COVID-19 pandemic.

2. Methods

2.1. Study Subjects

Schools in China were closed between January and May, 2020 due to the COVID-19 pandemic. An anonymous online survey was conducted to collect school-age children's responses regarding their background information, time use, and vision condition during this period of pandemic-led school closure. The questionnaire was distributed from 12 to 18 May 2020 via a nationally known education press, which solicited respondents from 29 provinces and autonomous regions. Completing the questionnaire takes about 10–15 min online. The inclusion criteria for participants were as follows: (1) literate and can understand the questionnaire; (2) enrolled in primary, lower-secondary, or upper-secondary schools; (3) voluntary participation; (4) submitted only one response using the same IP address; (5) whose guardian has submitted informed consent. A total of 3405 respondents from 1st to 12th grade satisfied the study's inclusion criteria. This study was approved by the Institutional Review Board of Shaanxi Normal University, and the study was conducted according to the World Medical Association Declaration of Helsinki.

2.2. Construct Measures

In order to facilitate the investigation, items on the questionnaire prompted respondents to self-evaluate symptomatic changes in their vision condition using the Lay Terms Approach, which advised using terminology that subjects are familiar with [22], such as "blurry vision when looking at distant objects" or "the need to squint." The standardized questionnaire also collected information on time (hours) spent using e-learning devices such as TVs, computers, or smartphones, and how frequent subjects engaged in outdoor exercise, as well as their subjective ratings of indoor lighting condition (too dim, too bright, or feels okay) while using e-learning devices. Following previous studies, we classified e-learning device use into three categories by device type—near (0.1 m for smartphones), intermediate (0.5 m for computers), and far (0.8 m for TVs)—and calculated daily digital screen use in diopter hours (dh), which is a viewing-distance weighted measure of near-vision exposure to digital devices [23].

dh = (3 × hours viewing at 0.1 m) + (2 × hours viewing at 0.5 m) + (1 × hours viewing at 0.8 m)

2.3. Statistical Analysis

In the first analytic step, we conducted univariate non-parametric analysis and reported chi-square test, as well as reporting parametric paired sample t-test results, in order to assess to what extent self-reported progression of myopic symptoms (dependent variable) differs by individual characteristics. A p-value of <0.05 was considered to be statistically significant. In the second analytic step, we fit multivariate logistic regression models to examine the association between digital screen use, outdoor activity, lighting condition, and self-reported myopia progression, after controlling for individual traits and pre-pandemic vision condition. The analyses were performed using STATA version 15.0 (Stata, StataCorp LLC, College Station, TX, USA) software.

3. Results

In Table 1, descriptive statistics of subject background information and results from the univariate nonparametric analysis are presented. Of the 3405 subjects that satisfied the inclusion criteria, 1358 (39.9%) reported myopic symptoms, 1647 (48.4%) were female, 2234 (65.6%) were in primary, 269 (7.9%) were in lower-secondary, and 902 (26.5%) were in upper-secondary schools, 540 (15.6%) were in rural areas, 248 (7.3%) were in urban–rural transitional areas, and 2627 (77.1%) were in urban cities. Among them, 1374 (40.4%) reported suffering from myopia prior to the COVID-19 pandemic. In terms of daily digital screen use, we first calculated daily digital screen use in diopter hours (dh), for which the sample mean is 10.0 diopter hours (SD = 6.3). We also reported daily digital screen use in unadjusted hours, which has a sample mean of 3.9 h (SD = 2.3). As for outdoor exercise, 620 (18.2%), 398 (11.7%), 1583 (46.5%), and 804 (23.6%) subjects reported as frequent, somewhat frequent, somewhat infrequent, and infrequent, respectively. For indoor lighting condition, 208 (6.1%) reported it being "too dim," 96 (2.8%) "too bright," and 3101 (91.1%) as "feels okay."

Table 1. Univariate parametric and nonparametric analysis.

Variable	Total (%)	Progression of Myopic Symptoms (Yes = 1, No = 0)		
		n	%	p
Progression of Myopic Symptoms				
Yes	39.9	-	-	-
No	60.1	-	-	-
Sex [a]				
Female	48.4	672	40.8	0.289
Male	51.6	686	39.0	
Grade of Enrolment [a]				
Primary	65.6	711	31.8	
Lower-Secondary	7.9	135	50.2	0.000
Upper-Secondary	26.5	512	56.8	
Location of Residence [a]				
Rural	15.6	196	37.0	
Urban–Rural	7.3	92	37.1	0.178
Urban	77.1	1070	40.7	
Pre-Pandemic Myopia Condition [a]				
Yes	40.4	806	58.7	0.000
No	59.6	552	27.2	
e-Learning Screen Use, diopter hours per day (mean, s.d., range) [b]	10.0, 6.3, 2–21	mean (1) − mean (0) = 3.7		0.000
e-Learning Screen Use, unadjusted hours per day (mean, s.d., range) [b]	3.9, 2.3, 1–10	mean (1) − mean (0) = 1.4		0.000
Outdoor Exercise [a]				
Frequent (daily)	18.2	250	40.3	
Somewhat Frequent (4–6 times/week)	11.7	132	33.2	0.000
Somewhat Infrequent (1–3 times/week)	46.5	588	37.2	
Infrequent (0 times/week)	23.6	388	48.3	
Indoor Lighting Condition [a]				
Too Dim	6.1	133	63.9	
Too Bright	2.8	55	57.3	0.000
Feels Okay	91.1	1170	37.7	

Notes: [a] p-value based on χ^2 test, [b] p-value based on t-test.

Under univariate nonparametric analysis, we examined the association between subject background characteristics, daily digital screen use, outdoor exercise, indoor lighting condition, and progression of myopic symptoms during the COVID-19 pandemic. First, myopic symptoms do not differ by subjects' sex ($\chi^2 = 1.124$, $p = 0.289$) or location of residence ($\chi^2 = 3.452$, $p = 0.178$). Second, subjects who reported myopic symptoms are more likely to be in lower-secondary and upper-secondary but less so in primary schools ($\chi^2 = 179.580$, $p < 0.001$). Third, subjects who suffer from a pre-pandemic myopia condition are also more likely to report symptomatic myopia progression during the COVID-19 pandemic ($\chi^2 = 338.785$, $p < 0.001$). Fourth, subjects who reported myopic symptoms on average engage in 3.7 more diopter hours than subjects who did not ($p < 0.001$). The same finding holds true without diopter adjustment, which is 1.4 unadjusted more so for subjects who reported myopic symptoms ($p < 0.001$). Fifth, subjects' frequency of participation in outdoor exercise is associated with the likelihood of reporting myopic symptoms ($\chi^2 = 36.015$, $p < 0.001$). Sixth, indoor lighting condition, particularly lighting condition that is too dim or too bright, is associated with progression of myopic symptoms ($\chi^2 = 68.347$, $p < 0.001$).

The distribution of the computed diopter hours result is displayed by enrolment level and by e-learning device type in Figure 1, from which two observations can be made. First, higher grade levels are associated with more intensive daily digital screen use in diopter hours. Second, smartphone is the most commonly used e-learning device reported across all grade levels.

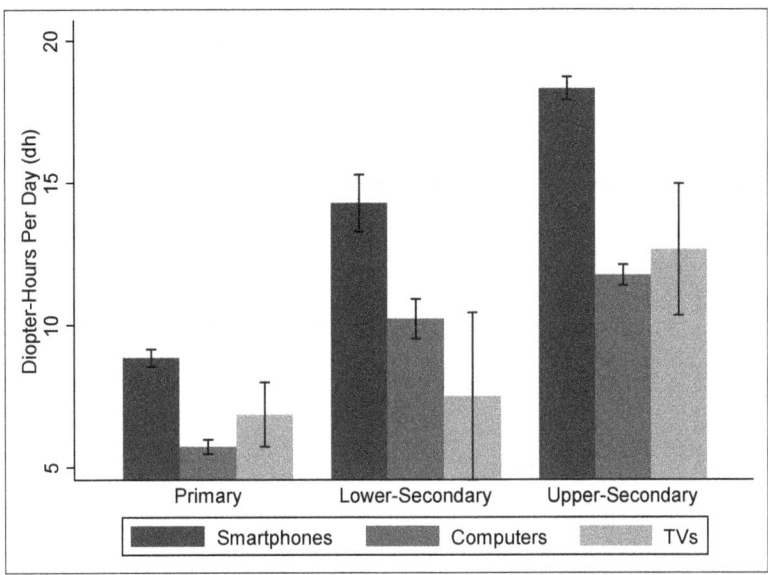

Figure 1. Daily use of e-learning devices among school-age children.

The multivariate logistic regression analysis was used to examine the association between e-learning screen use, outdoor activity, lighting condition, and myopia development, after adjusting for subjects' sex, grade, and location. Most strikingly, findings in Table 2 indicate that every diopter hour increase in daily e-learning screen use is significantly associated with progression of myopia symptoms (OR: 1.074, 95% CI: 1.058–1.089; $p < 0.001$). Since the sample average of daily digital screen use is 10.0 diopter hours, this result would imply substantial risks of myopic progression for the typical subject. In addition, subjects who engage in four to six times (OR: 0.745, 95% CI: 0.568–0.977; $p = 0.034$) and one to three times (OR: 0.829, 95% CI: 0.686–0.991; $p = 0.048$) of outdoor exercise per week are significantly less likely to report myopia symptoms than subjects who have no outdoor exercise each week. Finally, indoor lighting that is "too dim" (OR: 1.686, 95% CI: 1.226–2.319; $p = 0.001$) or "too bright" (OR: 1.529, 95% CI: 1.007–2.366; $p = 0.036$) is significantly associated with a higher likelihood of myopia symptoms, relative to the comfortable indoor lighting condition. The association between pre-pandemic myopia condition and progression of myopia symptoms is also statistically significant (OR: 2.814, 95% CI: 2.376–3.334; $p < 0.001$).

Table 2. Multivariate logistic regression analysis.

Variables	Progression of Myopic Symptoms (Yes = 1, No = 0)		
	OR	95% CI	p
e-Learning Screen Use, diopter hours per day (dh)	1.074	1.058–1.089	0.000
Outdoor Exercise			
Frequent (daily)	0.994	0.788–1.255	0.962
Somewhat Frequent (4–6 times/week)	0.745	0.568–0.977	0.034
Somewhat Infrequent (1–3 times/week)	0.829	0.686–0.991	0.048
Infrequent (0 times/week)	1		
Indoor Lighting Condition			
Too Dim	1.686	1.226–2.319	0.001
Too Bright	1.529	1.007–2.366	0.036
Feels Okay	1		
Sex			
Female	0.990	0.853–1.149	0.895
Male	1		
Grade of Enrolment			
Primary	1.006	0.756–1.340	0.966
Lower-Secondary	0.907	0.676–1.217	0.514
Upper-Secondary	1		
Location of Residence			
Rural	0.988	0.801–1.220	0.913
Urban–Rural	0.872	0.651–1.167	0.514
Urban	1		
Pre-Pandemic Myopia Condition			
Yes	2.814	2.376–3.334	0.000
No	1		

Notes: OR = odds ratio; CI = confidence interval.

4. Discussion

A substantial portion of primary and secondary schools in China were closed between January and May of 2020, and a majority of school-age children had to resort to online e-learning using computers, smartphones, or TVs. Importantly, these remote learning arrangements may present new risk factors for youth vision development as a consequence of changes in daily physical and eye-use behavior among children. To the best of our knowledge, this study is one of the first to examine the association between digital screen use, outdoor activity, lighting condition, and myopia development among school-age children in the context of a nationwide remote learning experiment during the COVID-19 outbreak in China.

Using a large-scale national survey, we presented three main findings. First, we found that the duration of daily digital screen use among school-age children during the COVID-19 outbreak in China is substantial, measuring at 3.9 h daily on average. Once weighting by viewing-distance is considered, near-vision exposure to digital devices rises to 10.0 diopter hours daily. Using multivariate logistic regression analysis, we found that each additional diopter hour of digital screen use is associated with a higher likelihood of symptomatic myopia development, which can translate into significant risks considering the extended periods of time young children spend in front of digital screens daily. Second, approximately one in four school-age children in our sample do not perform any outdoor exercise during the COVID-19 school closures, and more than 70 percent engage in outdoor exercise less than three times per week. Prior studies have highlighted the positive influence outdoor playtime can have on visual acuity as well as the associated health risks the lackthereof [7]. In our analysis, we found that more frequent outdoor exercise is generally associated with a lower likelihood of myopia development. Third, approximately one in ten school-age children in our sample report that indoor lighting condition is either too dim or too bright at home. As the main venue for learning activities during the COVID-19 pandemic, indoor lighting conditions critically affect children's vision development, and poor lighting conditions are associated with a higher likelihood of worsening vision status among children in the study sample.

We contribute to the current literature on youth public health and build on prior studies on adolescent health that examine the association between near-vision electronic use [24], outdoor activity [7], lighting condition [21], and myopic vision progression by assessing these risk factors in conjunction and leveraging an extended period of COVID-19-pandemic-induced remote learning. While this study does not directly assess how student learning is affected, prior studies have underscored the critical negative impact myopic vision can have on student learning, particularly if corrective vision interventions are not afforded [25]. In this regard, our findings tend to confirm speculative predictions of a myopia boom during the COVID-19 pandemic [3] and are consistent with a recent longitudinal study on Chinese youth that indicated the positive association between digital screen exposure and prevalence of myopia [26] while complementing a recent cross-sectional study that examined how home confinement can have adverse effects on youth vision health [27], with richer information on digital screen use and indoor lighting condition. Based on our findings, we speculate that extended periods of school closure due to public health crises, such as the COVID-19 pandemic, and consequent alternative learning arrangements at home can increase the risks of inducing a myopia boom among school-age children. However, mitigation strategies such as limiting near-vision digital screen use duration, increasing outdoor exercise frequency, and improving indoor lighting conditions may prove to be effective in reducing, or delaying, such a youth visual health crisis [28]. While these findings are context-specific to school-age youth in China, the broader behavioral and policy implications are broadly relevant for a wide range of countries whose education system is making or is expecting to implement similar e-learning accommodations during the COVID-19 pandemic.

Finally, a limitation in this study worth mentioning is relying on subjects' self-reports rather than specialist eye examinations. While professional ophthalmic evaluations would be ideal to obtain detailed information on refractive error, prior studies have suggested that subjects' self-assessment of vision status does not differ systemically from professional ophthalmic evaluations [29]. Additionally, another reason for adopting self-reported measures is to allow for rapid and large-scale survey rollout [30], which would not have been feasible given the logistical and social-distancing requirements due to the COVID-19 pandemic. Nonetheless, it has been increasingly common in optometry and visual science studies to leverage questionnaire survey designs, considering the relatively high cost-effectiveness [24]. Future studies may find it useful to conduct professional ophthalmic evaluations in lieu of collecting subject self-reports.

5. Conclusions

The public health consequences stemming from a pandemic can be both wide-ranging and long-lasting, affecting not only the most vulnerable, but also leave its mark on the next generation in profound ways. In this study, we identified the less-visible vision health concerns on young children as many education systems have transitioned to remote online instruction due to the COVID-19 pandemic. Most strikingly, near-vision e-learning device use is a critical source affecting myopia development, and the associated youth health risks, as well as appropriate mitigation strategies, need to be seriously considered, should remote learning programs continue due to prolonged future waves of the COVID-19 pandemic.

Author Contributions: J.L., Q.C., and J.D. conceived, conceptualized, and designed the study. J.L. and Q.C. contributed to data collection and conducted the statistical analysis. J.L., B.L., and Q.C. drafted the article and contributed to interpretation of results. All authors have revised the manuscript for important intellectual content. All authors have read and agreed to the published version of the manuscript.

Funding: This work was supported by the National Social Science Foundation of China (CJA200256) and Shaanxi Normal University RenCai Faculty Seed Fund (1301031829).

Institutional Review Board Statement: The study was conducted according to the guidelines of the Declaration of Helsinki and approved by the Institutional Review Board (76909767).

Informed Consent Statement: All subject consent was obtained.

Data Availability Statement: Restrictions apply to the availability of data used, due to study subject privacy protection. Data was obtained from Teachers Daily and is available upon request with the permission of Teachers Daily.

Acknowledgments: We thank Xiangna Kong and Xiaoli Feng at Teachers Daily for data collaboration.

Conflicts of Interest: The authors have no conflicts of interest to disclose.

References

1. UNESCO. *How Many Students Are at Risk of not Returning to School?* UNESCO: Paris, France, 2020.
2. CGDEV. *COVID-19 Education Policy Tracker*; Center for Global Development: Washington, DC, USA, 2020.
3. Wong, C.W.; Tsai, A.; Jonas, J.B.; Ohno-Matsui, K.; Chen, J.; Ang, M.; Ting, D.S.W. Digital Screen Time During the COVID-19 Pandemic: Risk for a Further Myopia Boom? *Am. J. Ophthalmol.* **2021**, *223*, 333–337. [CrossRef]
4. Navel, V.; Beze, S.; Dutheil, F. COVID-19, sweat, tears ... and myopia? *Clin. Exp. Optom.* **2020**, *103*, 555. [CrossRef]
5. Holden, B.A.; Fricke, T.R.; Wilson, D.A.; Jong, M.; Naidoo, K.S.; Sankaridurg, P.; Wong, T.Y.; Naduvilath, T.J.; Resnikoff, S. Global Prevalence of Myopia and High Myopia and Temporal Trends from 2000 through 2050. *Ophthalmology.* **2016**, *123*, 1036–1042. [CrossRef]
6. Smith, E.L.; Hung, L.-F.; Arumugam, B. Visual regulation of refractive development: Insights from animal studies. *Eye* **2014**, *28*, 180–188. [CrossRef]
7. Guan, H.; Yu, N.N.; Wang, H.; Boswell, M.; Shi, Y.; Rozelle, S.; Congdon, N. Impact of various types of near work and time spent outdoors at different times of day on visual acuity and refractive error among Chinese school-going children. *PLoS ONE* **2019**, *14*, e0215827. [CrossRef] [PubMed]
8. Regan, A.; Arne, O.; Frank, S. The Effect of Ambient Illuminance on the Development of Deprivation Myopia in Chicks. *Investig. Ophthalmol. Vis. Sci.* **2009**, *50*, 5348–5354.
9. Saw, S.-M.; Matsumura, S.; Hoang, Q.V. Prevention and Management of Myopia and Myopic Pathology. *Investig. Opthalmol. Vis. Sci.* **2019**, *60*, 488–499. [CrossRef] [PubMed]
10. Leo, S.W.; Young, T.L. An evidence-based update on myopia and interventions to retard its progression. *J. Am. Assoc. Pediatr. Ophthalmol. Strabismus* **2011**, *15*, 181–189. [CrossRef] [PubMed]
11. Saw, S.-M.; Gazzard, G.; Shih-Yen, E.C.; Chua, W.-H. Myopia and associated pathological complications. *Ophthalmic Physiol. Opt.* **2005**, *25*, 381–391. [CrossRef]
12. Tideman, J.W.L.; Snabel, M.C.; Tedja, M.S.; Van Rijn, G.A.; Wong, K.T.; Kuijpers, R.W.; Vingerling, J.R.; Hofman, A.; Buitendijk, G.H.S.; Keunen, J.E.E.; et al. Association of Axial Length with Risk of Uncorrectable Visual Impairment for Eu-ropeans With Myopia. *JAMA Ophthalmol.* **2016**, *134*, 1355–1363. [CrossRef] [PubMed]
13. Morgan, I.G.; Ohno-Matsui, K.; Saw, S.M. Myopia. *Lancet* **2012**, *379*, 1739–1748. [CrossRef]
14. Theophanous, C.; Modjtahedi, B.S.; Batech, M.; Marlin, D.S.; Luong, T.Q.; Fong, D.S. Myopia prevalence and risk factors in children. *Clin. Ophthalmol.* **2018**, *12*, 1581–1587. [CrossRef]
15. He, M.; Zheng, Y.; Xiang, F. Prevalence of Myopia in Urban and Rural Children in Mainland China. *Optom. Vis. Sci.* **2009**, *86*, 40–44. [CrossRef]
16. Chua, S.Y.; Sabanayagam, C.; Cheung, Y.B.; Chia, A.; Valenzuela, R.K.; Tan, D.; Wong, T.-Y.; Cheng, C.-Y.; Saw, S.M. Age of onset of myopia predicts risk of high myopia in later childhood in myop-ic Singapore children. *Ophthalmic Physiol. Opt.* **2016**, *36*, 388–394. [CrossRef] [PubMed]
17. Smith, E.L.; Hung, L.-F.; Huang, J. Relative peripheral hyperopic defocus alters central refractive development in infant monkeys. *Vis. Res.* **2009**, *49*, 2386–2392. [CrossRef]
18. Long, J.; Cheung, R.; Duong, S.; Paynter, R.; Asper, L. Viewing distance and eyestrain symptoms with prolonged viewing of smartphones. *Clin. Exp. Optom.* **2017**, *100*, 133–137. [CrossRef] [PubMed]
19. Narimatsu, T.; Negishi, K.; Miyake, S.; Hirasawa, M.; Osada, H.; Kurihara, T.; Tsubota, K.; Ozawa, Y. Blue light-induced inflammatory marker expression in the retinal pigment epithe-lium-choroid of mice and the protective effect of a yellow intraocular lens material in vivo. *Exp. Eye Res.* **2015**, *132*, 48–51. [CrossRef]
20. Flitcroft, D. The complex interactions of retinal, optical and environmental factors in myopia aetiology. *Prog. Retin. Eye Res.* **2012**, *31*, 622–660. [CrossRef] [PubMed]
21. Ashby, R. Animal Studies and the Mechanism of Myopia—Protection by Light? *Optom. Vis. Sci.* **2016**, *93*, 1052–1054. [CrossRef]
22. Walline, J.J.; Zadnik, K.; Mutti, D.O. Validity of Surveys Reporting Myopia, Astigmatism, and Presbyopia. *Optom. Vis. Sci.* **1996**, *73*, 376–381. [CrossRef]

23. Williams, R.; Bakshi, S.; Ostrin, E.J.; Ostrin, L.A. Continuous Objective Assessment of Near Work. *Sci. Rep.* **2019**, *9*, 1–10. [CrossRef]
24. Talens-Estarelles, C.; Sanchis-Jurado, V.; Esteve-Taboada, J.J.; Pons, Á.M.; García-Lázaro, S. How Do Different Digital Displays Affect the Ocular Surface? *Optom. Vis. Sci.* **2020**, *97*, 1070–1079. [CrossRef] [PubMed]
25. Jan, C.L.; Timbo, C.S.; Congdon, N. Children's myopia: Prevention and the role of school programmes. *Community Eye Health* **2017**, *30*, 37–38. [PubMed]
26. Yang, G.-Y.; Huang, L.-H.; Schmid, K.L.; Li, C.-G.; Chen, J.-Y.; He, G.-H.; Liu, L.; Ruan, Z.-L.; Chen, W.-Q. Associations between Screen Exposure in Early Life and Myopia amongst Chinese Preschoolers. *Int. J. Environ. Res. Public Health* **2020**, *17*, 1056. [CrossRef] [PubMed]
27. Wang, J.; Li, Y.; Musch, D.C.; Wei, N.; Qi, X.; Ding, G.; Li, X.; Li, J.; Song, L.; Zhang, Y.; et al. Progression of Myopia in School-Aged Children After COVID-19 Home Confinement. *JAMA Ophthalmol.* **2021**, *139*, 293. [CrossRef]
28. Wang, G.; Zhang, Y.; Zhao, J.; Zhang, J.; Jiang, F. Mitigate the effects of home confinement on children during the COVID-19 outbreak. *Lancet* **2020**, *395*, 945–947. [CrossRef]
29. Cumberland, P.M.; Chianca, A.; Rahi, J. Accuracy and Utility of Self-report of Refractive Error. *JAMA Ophthalmol.* **2016**, *134*, 794–801. [CrossRef] [PubMed]
30. McFadden, P.; Ross, J.; Moriarty, J.; Mallett, J.; Schroder, H.; Ravalier, J.; Manthorpe, J.; Currie, D.; Harron, J.; Gillen, P. The Role of Coping in the Wellbeing and Work-Related Quality of Life of UK Health and Social Care Workers during COVID-19. *Int. J. Environ. Res. Public Health* **2021**, *18*, 815. [CrossRef]

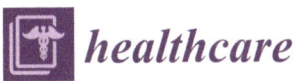

Article

Postponed Dental Visits during the COVID-19 Pandemic and their Correlates. Evidence from the Nationally Representative COVID-19 Snapshot Monitoring in Germany (COSMO)

André Hajek [1,*], Freia De Bock [2], Lena Huebl [3], Benedikt Kretzler [1] and Hans-Helmut König [1]

1. Department of Health Economics and Health Services Research, Hamburg Center for Health Economics, University Medical Center Hamburg-Eppendorf, 20251 Hamburg, Germany; b.kretzler.ext@uke.de (B.K.); h.koenig@uke.de (H.-H.K.)
2. Federal Centre of Health Education, 50825 Cologne, Germany; freia.debock@bzga.de
3. Department of Tropical Medicine, Bernhard Nocht Institute for Tropical Medicine, University Medical Center Hamburg-Eppendorf, 20251 Hamburg, Germany; l.huebl@uke.de
* Correspondence: a.hajek@uke.de

Citation: Hajek, A.; De Bock, F.; Huebl, L.; Kretzler, B.; König, H.-H. Postponed Dental Visits during the COVID-19 Pandemic and their Correlates. Evidence from the Nationally Representative COVID-19 Snapshot Monitoring in Germany (COSMO). *Healthcare* **2021**, *9*, 50. https://doi.org/10.3390/healthcare9010050

Received: 4 December 2020
Accepted: 28 December 2020
Published: 5 January 2021

Publisher's Note: MDPI stays neutral with regard to jurisdictional clai-ms in published maps and institutio-nal affiliations.

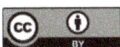

Copyright: © 2021 by the authors. Licensee MDPI, Basel, Switzerland. This article is an open access article distributed under the terms and conditions of the Creative Commons Attribution (CC BY) license (https://creativecommons.org/licenses/by/4.0/).

Abstract: (1) Background: The COVID-19 pandemic is accompanied by various societal and economic challenges. Furthermore, it is associated with major health challenges. Oral health is a key component of health. Therefore, both curative and preventive dental visits are important during pandemics. Since there is a lack of nationally representative studies focusing on postponed dental visits and their correlates during the COVID-19 pandemic, we aimed to fill this gap in knowledge; (2) Methods: Cross-sectional data (wave 17) were collected from a nationally representative online-survey (COVID-19 Snapshot Monitoring in Germany (COSMO)) conducted in July 2020. The analytical sample consisted of 974 individuals (average age was 45.9 years (SD: 16.5, from 18 to 74 years)). The outcome measure was postponed dental visits since March 2020 (yes; no) due to the COVID-19 pandemic. Furthermore, the type of postponed dental visits was recorded (check-up/regular dental examination; pain/dental complaints; planned therapy); (3) Results: 22% of participants reported to have postponed dental visits due to the COVID-19 pandemic since March 2020, whereas 78% of individuals did not report postponed visits ("no, attended as planned": 29.2%; "no, examining pending": 44.9%; "no, other reasons": 3.9%). Among individuals who reported postponed dental visits, 72% postponed a "check-up/regular dental examination", whereas 8.4% postponed a dental visit despite "pain/dental complaints" and 19.6% postponed "planned therapy". Furthermore, multiple logistic regressions showed that the likelihood of postponed dental visits was positively associated with being younger (aged 65 and older, OR: 0.43, 95% CI: 0.22–0.85; compared to individuals 18 to 29 years), and higher affect regarding COVID-19 (OR: 1.36, 95% CI: 1.13–1.64); (4) Conclusions: Our study showed that more than one out of five individuals postponed a dental visit—particularly check-ups and regular dental examination—due to the COVID-19 pandemic since March 2020. Several correlates of these postponed visits have been identified. This may help identify and address individuals at risk for deterioration of oral health amplified by postponed dental visits.

Keywords: COVID-19; coronavirus; dental care; dental health services; dental visits; SARS-CoV-2; dental service use; postponed dental visits; check-up; dental examination; pain; dental complaints; oral health

1. Introduction

Access to regular dental visits is important to avoiding oral diseases [1,2]. Nevertheless, it should be noted that avoiding or postponing dental visits is frequent in Germany [3,4]. For example, this behavior could lead to periodontitis and caries lesions which could ultimately result in tooth loos [5]. Furthermore, postponed dental visits can additionally affect quality of life [6]. Consequently, poor oral health can decrease functional health [7].

Previous studies have focused on determinants of nonattendance and dental treatment avoidance [4,8], rather than postponement of dental visits as the outcome measure. Furthermore, studies determined postponement for financial reasons [3]. For example, it has been shown that dental anxiety is associated with avoidance behavior [8]. Moreover, it has been demonstrated that avoidance of dental treatment is associated with younger age, lower social status, unemployment, and decreased health (in terms of increased physical illnesses and increased depressive symptoms) [4].

Existing studies focused on nonattendance, avoidance, or postponement of dental visits prior to the COVID-19 pandemic. Thus far, one economic analysis using a modelling approach exists focusing on the impact of COVID-19 on dental practices [9]. A telephone-based survey conducted from 24 March to 2 April 2020 (146 German dentists) [9] showed that mitigation/suppression decreased use of dental services, particularly prevention (−80% in mean), periodontics (−76%), and prosthetics (−70%). According to Schwendicke et al., COVID-19 and associated policies had an economic impact on dental practices in Germany [9]. Comparably, a study conducted in China (Beijing) from 1 February to 10 February 2020 showed that the COVID-19 pandemic significantly decreased the use of emergency dental services (e.g., 38% fewer patients had emergency dental visits at the beginning of the COVID-19 pandemic compared to one month prior to the pandemic) [10]. During the same period, the proportion of oral and dental infections significantly increased [10].

However, up to now, nationally representative studies focusing on postponed dental visits (in general, rather than directly cost-related) and its correlates are lacking. We aimed to fill this gap in knowledge.

To put our findings into context, in Germany, corona measures such as school closings or closing of daycare centers were implemented on 16 March 2020. A week later (22 March 2020), public restrictions and travel bans followed. These measures were prolonged in subsequent weeks. Restrictions were loosened on the 20 April 2020. In the beginning of May, schools gradually reopened. In May, additional restrictions were loosened (e.g., playgrounds reopened and contact bans loosened). Further restrictions eased in June. Nevertheless, a spike in COVID-19 cases could lead to a reimplementation of regulations.

It is necessary to describe key characteristics of the German healthcare system. Health insurance is compulsory in Germany. Approximately 9 out of 10 individuals are members of the social statutory health insurance (SHI), solely 1 out of 10 individuals has private health insurance (PHI). Predominantly, civil servants, employed individuals exceeding a defined income threshold, and self-employed individuals can opt for PHI. Both categories of health insurance (PHI and SHI) cover most expenses of outpatient treatment (even for dental care services) in Germany. Access to health care is commonly guaranteed for all insured individuals. However, additional dental services (e.g., gold or ceramic inlays) which have an unproven medical benefit are usually not covered in SHI. It should be emphasized that waiting periods are relatively short in Germany [11,12]. Passon et al. give further insight into the German health care system [13]. With regard to the COVID-19 pandemic, it should be noted that routine dentistry was allowed to continue in Germany. It was therefore not restricted to emergency appointments.

2. Materials and Methods

2.1. Sample

Cross-sectional data were collected from wave 17 of the COVID-19 Snapshot Monitoring (COSMO) [14]. Solely in wave 17 individuals were asked about postponed dental visits.

The COSMO study started in early March 2020 (3rd/4th March) with weekly follow-up waves until 26 May. Afterwards, the survey continued in a 14-day interval. Wave 17 was conducted from 21st to 22nd of July 2020. In wave 17, n = 1001 individuals aged 18 to 74 years participated. Individuals younger than 18 years and individuals older than 74 years were excluded in this wave.

A market research company (Respondi) conducted the recruitment of participants from an online panel matching distribution of age, gender (crossed-quota: age x gender), and federal state (uncrossed) within the German population [15]. A large sample size was chosen to also detect small effects in the COSMO study [16].

Informed consent was obtained from all individual participants included in the study. Ethical approval for COSMO was obtained by University of Erfurt's IRB (#202000302). All procedures performed in the COSMO studies involving human participants were in accordance with the ethical standards of the University of Erfurt institutional research committee and with the 1964 Helsinki Declaration and its later amendments or comparable ethical standards.

2.2. Dependent Variables

In concordance to other large cohort studies (e.g., Survey of Health, Ageing, and Retirement in Europe) individuals were first asked whether they had postponed a dental visit since March 2020 due to the COVID-19 pandemic (1 "Yes", 2 "No, attended as planned", 3 "No examination pending", 4 "No, other reasons"). The outcome measure was dichotomized (0 = no, not postponed; 1= yes, postponed). Additionally, individuals were asked about the type of postponed dental visit (1 = "check-up/regular dental examination", 2 = "pain/dental complaints", and 3 = "planned therapy").

A pretest with $n = 14$ individuals confirmed high face validity of our outcome measures.

2.3. Independent Variables

Various determinants were included in our study: sex, age group (distinguishing between: 18 to 29 years; 30 to 49 years; 50 to 64 years; 65 years and above), relationship/marriage (no; yes), presence of children under 18 years (no; yes), living arrangement (two or more individuals in the same household; living alone), migration background (no; yes), status of self-employment (no; yes), educational level (up to 9 years/10 years and more (without general qualification for university entrance); 10 years and more (with general qualification for university entrance)), region (East Germany; West Germany), town size (municipality/small town (1–20,000); medium sized town (20,001–100,000); small city (100,001–500,000); big city (>500,000)), COVID-19 cases/100,000 population (below median; above median), and chronic diseases (no; yes).

With regard to COVID-19, individuals were asked to rate how they were affected (consisting of seven items, seven-point scale). For instance, items were: "For me, the new type of corona virus is" ... "near" (1) to "far away" (7) or "inflated in media" (1) to "not given enough attention in media" (7) or "Something I keep thinking about" (1) to "Something I almost never think about" (7).

The total score was built by averaging items. In our study, Cronbach's alpha was 0.78. Moreover, participants were asked to rate the severity of COVID-19 disease ("How do you assess an infection with the novel corona virus for yourself?", from 1 = completely harmless to 7 = extremely dangerous).

2.4. Statistical Analysis

Sample characteristics (analytical sample) were first calculated stratified by postponement of dental visits (no; yes). Afterwards, multiple logistic regressions were performed to identify determinants of postponed dental visits due to the COVID-19 pandemic. In further analysis, we used a multinomial logistic regression (with "Yes, postponed dental visits" as the base outcome). Statistical significance was set at $p < 0.05$. p values between 0.05 and 0.10 were considered as marginally significant. Statistical analyses were performed using Stata 16.0 (Stata Corp., College Station, TX, USA).

3. Results

3.1. Sample Characteristics

Sample characteristics for our analytical sample ($n = 974$) are shown in Table 1. In the total sample, the average age equaled 45.9 years (SD: 16.5, from 18 to 74 years) with 51.1% of individuals being female. Postponed dental visits were associated with being female, age category, and affect regarding COVID-19. Further details are shown in Table 1.

Table 1. Sample characteristics for the analytical sample (n = 974 individuals) at wave 17.

Independent Variables	Postponed Dental Visits				p-Value
	Yes, Postponed Dental Visits Mean (SD)/n (%)	No, Attended as Planned Mean (SD)/n (%)	No Examining Pending Mean (SD)/n (%)	No, other Reasons Mean (SD)/n (%)	
Sex					<0.01
Men	91 (19.1%)	127 (26.7%)	240 (50.4%)	18 (3.8%)	
Women	123 (24.7%)	158 (31.7%)	197 (39.6%)	20 (4.0%)	
Age category					<0.01
18 to 29 years	36 (19.1%)	63 (33.3)	83 (43.9%)	7 (3.7)	
30 to 49 years	102 (29.1%)	92 (26.3%)	140 (40.0%)	16 (4.6%)	
50 to 64 years	57 (21.1%)	78 (28.9%)	124 (45.9%)	11 (4.1%)	
65 years and over	19 (11.5%)	52 (31.5%)	90 (54.6%)	4 (2.4%)	
Children under 18 years:					0.07
No	145 (20.1%)	219 (30.3%)	332 (46.0%)	26 (3.6%)	
Yes	69 (27.4%)	66 (26.2%)	105 (41.7%)	12 (4.7%)	
Education					0.53
up to 9 years/10 years and more (without general qualification for university entrance)	88 (19.9%)	132 (29.8%)	206 (46.5%)	17 (3.8%)	
10 years and more (with general qualification for university entrance)	126 (23.7%)	153 (28.8%)	231 (43.5%)	21 (4.0)	
Town size					0.34
Municipality/small town (1–20.000)	80 (19.9%)	128 (31.8%)	174 (43.3%)	20 (5.0%)	
Medium sized town (20.001–100.000)	53 (22.1%)	68 (28.3%)	115 (47.9%)	4 (1.7%)	
Small city (100.001–500.000)	30 (21.1%)	40 (28.2%)	65 (45.8%)	7 (4.9%)	
Big city (> 500.000)	51 (26.8%)	49 (25.8%)	83 (43.7%)	7 (3.7%)	
Region					0.10
West Germany	181 (22.2%)	229 (28.0%)	371 (45.4%)	36 (4.4%)	
East Germany	33 (21.0%)	56 (35.7%)	66 (42.0%)	2 (1.3%)	
Cases/100,000 population					0.40
Below median	109 (23.3%)	142 (30.3%)	197 (42.1%)	20 (4.3%)	
Above median	105 (20.8%)	143 (28.3%)	240 (47.4%)	18 (3.6%)	
Relationship/Marriage					0.35
No	66 (19.6%)	103 (30.5%)	158 (46.9%)	10 (3.0%)	
Yes	148 (23.2%)	182 (28.6%)	279 (43.8%)	28 (4.4%)	
Living situation					0.85
Living alone	54 (21.3%)	73 (28.9%)	118 (46.6%)	8 (3.2%)	
At least 2 individuals in the same household	160 (22.2%)	212 (29.4%)	319 (44.2%)	30 (4.2%)	
Migration background:					0.82
No	183 (22.2%)	236 (28.7%)	372 (45.2%)	32 (3.9%)	
Yes	31 (20.5%)	49 (32.4%)	65 (43.1%)	6 (4.0%)	
Self-employment					0.50
No	196 (22.2%)	252 (28.5%)	400 (45.3%)	35 (4.0%)	
Yes	18 (19.8%)	33 (36.3%)	37 (40.6%)	3 (3.3%)	
Chronic disease					0.20
No	127 (20.9%)	187 (30.7%)	276 (45.3%)	19 (3.1%)	
Yes	87 (23.8%)	98 (26.9%)	161 (44.1%)	19 (5.2%)	

Table 1. Cont.

Independent Variables	Yes, Postponed Dental Visits Mean (SD)/n (%)	Postponed Dental Visits		No, other Reasons Mean (SD)/n (%)	p-Value
		No, Attended as Planned Mean (SD)/n (%)	No Examining Pending Mean (SD)/n (%)		
Affect regarding COVID-19 (higher values correspond to higher affect regarding COVID-19)	4.4 (1.0)	4.1 (0.9)	4.1 (1.1)	4.2 (1.1)	<0.001
Presumed severity of COVID-19 infection (from 1 to 7; higher values correspond to higher severity)	4.4 (1.6)	4.1 (1.5)	4.1 (1.6)	4.3 (1.7)	0.09

In sum, 22% of participants reported to have postponed dental visits due to the COVID-19 pandemic since March 2020, 78% did not report postponed visits ("no, attended as planned: 29.2%; "no, examining pending": 44.9%; "no, other reasons": 3.9%), as shown in Figure 1. Of the individuals who reported postponed dental visits, 72% postponed a "check-up/regular dental examination", whereas 8.4% postponed a dental visit despite "pain/dental complaints" and 19.6% postponed "planned therapy" (Figure 2).

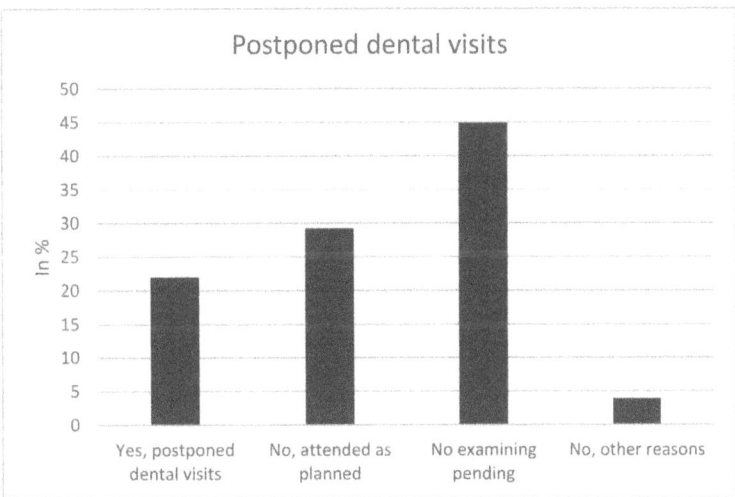

Figure 1. Postponed dental visits.

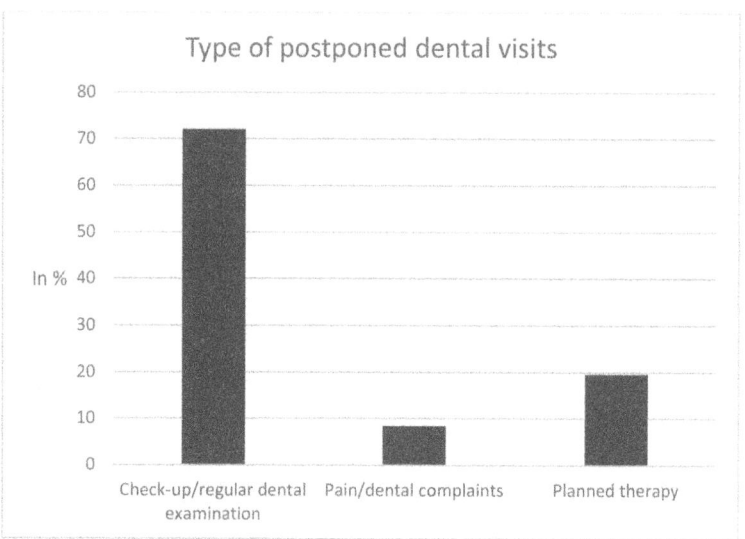

Figure 2. Type of postponed dental visits.

3.2. Regression Analysis

Multiple logistic regressions with postponed dental visits (0 = no, not postponed; 1 = yes, postponed) as outcome measures are displayed in Table 2. Regressions revealed that the likelihood of postponed dental visits due to the COVID-19 pandemic since March 2020 was positively associated with being younger (aged 65 and older, OR: 0.43, 95% CI: 0.22–0.85; compared to individuals 18 to 29 years), and higher affect regarding COVID-19 (OR: 1.36, 95% CI: 1.13–1.64). Furthermore, there was a marginal significant positive association between postponed dental visits and big cities (compared to small towns, OR: 1.53, 95% CI: 0.99–2.34). The remaining variables were not significantly associated with the outcome measure.

The results of further analysis with multinomial logistic regression (with "Yes, postponed dental visits" as the base outcome) are displayed in Supplementary Table S1. Findings remained comparable to our findings using multiple logistic regressions.

Table 2. Determinants of postponed dental visits (0 – no, not postponed; 1 = yes, postponed) due to the COVID-19 pandemic since March 2020. Findings of multiple logistic regressions.

Independent Variables	Postponed Dental Visits
Gender: Female (Ref.: Male)	1.30
	(0.95–1.79)
Age category: 30 to 49 years (Ref.: 18 to 29 years)	1.42
	(0.87–2.32)
50 to 64 years	0.96
	(0.56–1.63)
65 years and over	0.43 *
	(0.22–0.85)
Children (under 18 years): Yes (Ref.: Absence of children under 18 years)	1.20
	(0.81–1.77)
Education: General qualification for university entrance (Ref.: absence of qualification for university entrance)	1.18
	(0.84–1.65)

Table 2. Cont.

Independent Variables	Postponed Dental Visits
Town size: Medium sized town (20,001–100,000) (Ref.: municipality/small town (1–20,000))	1.16
	(0.77–1.74)
Small city (100,001–500,000)	1.09
	(0.67–1.80)
Big city (> 500,000)	1.53 +
	(0.99–2.34)
Region: East Germany (Ref.: West Germany)	0.84
	(0.52–1.35)
Cases/100,000 population: Above median (Ref.: below median)	0.82
	(0.58–1.17)
Relationship/Marriage: Yes (Ref.: no partnership/marriage)	1.17
	(0.76–1.80)
Living situation: At least 2 individuals in the same household (Ref.: living alone)	0.92
	(0.57–1.47)
Migration background: Yes (Ref.: no migration background)	0.85
	(0.54–1.36)
Self-employment: Yes (Ref.: not self-employed)	0.79
	(0.45–1.39)
Chronic disease: Yes (Ref.: no chronic diseases)	1.14
	(0.81–1.61)
Affect: COVID-19 infection (higher values correspond to higher affect)	1.36 **
	(1.13–1.64)
Severity: COVID-19 infection (higher values correspond to higher severity)	1.07
	(0.94–1.22)
Constant	0.04 ***
	(0.01–0.14)
Observations	974
R^2	0.06

Odds ratios are reported; 95% confidence intervals in parentheses; *** $p < 0.001$, ** $p < 0.01$, * $p < 0.05$, + $p < 0.10$.

4. Discussion

Based on nationally representative cross-sectional data, the aim of this study was to clarify the frequency of postponed dental visits due to the COVID-19 pandemic and to determine its associated factors. Furthermore, the type of postponed dental visits was displayed (check-up/regular dental examination; pain/dental complaints; planned therapy). Based on individuals who postponed dental visits or did not attend as planned, it should be emphasized that approximately 43% of individuals postponed dental visits, and a significant amount postponed dental visits despite "pain/dental complaints". Our study extends previous knowledge focusing on actual use of dental services in early 2020 [10] or modeled use of dental services [9].

Our study showed that more than one out of five individuals postponed a dental visit due to the COVID-19 pandemic between March and July 2020, particularly check-ups and regular dental examination. Predominantly individuals aged 30 to 49 years (29.1%) postponed dental visits. Regressions revealed that the likelihood of postponed dental visits was positively associated with being younger and higher affect regarding COVID-19.

Younger individuals are at an increased risk of postponing dental visits because they have to fulfill family and job obligations concurrently (e.g., compared to older adults, 65 years and above). The burden increased during the COVID-19 pandemic due to, e.g., school closings and the requirement to work from home. Furthermore, the link between increased affect regarding COVID-19 and postponed dental visits appears plausible. Previous studies have shown a link between dental fear and avoidance of dental visits [17]. It should be noted that (negative) affect is commonly associated with fear or anxiety-related factors [18]. Since there was a lack of studies quantifying the reasons for postponed dental visits, it was difficult to compare our results with studies published in past years.

Postponing dental visits can have serious consequences for oral health. For example, it could result in caries lesions and periodontitis which, in turn, could increase the likelihood of tooth loos [5] or dental pain [19]. This is important, since the COVID-19 pandemic can markedly affect oral health [20–22]. Even in the light of the effect of different recall intervals [23], our current findings are therefore of great importance.

This is the first study showing the frequency and correlates of postponed dental visits in Germany during the COVID-19 pandemic. Another strength is that nationally representative data were used. Additionally, the type of postponed dental visits was recorded. One limitation is its cross-sectional design with the acknowledged limitations. Future research is needed to examine postponed dental visits among individuals aged 75 years and older. Moreover, future research is required to explicitly clarify whether the postponed dental visits were postponed by the patient or by the clinician. Furthermore, upcoming studies should include factors such as dental anxiety.

5. Conclusions

In conclusion, data showed that more than one out of five individuals postponed a dental visit—particularly check-ups and regular dental examination—due to the COVID-19 pandemic between March and July 2020. Some determinants of these postponed visits have been identified, namely age and affect regarding COVID-19. The findings may help identify and address individuals at risk for deterioration of oral health due to postponed dental visits.

Supplementary Materials: The following are available online at https://www.mdpi.com/2227-9032/9/1/50/s1, Table S1: Determinants of postponed dental visits due to the COVID-19 pandemic since March 2020. Findings of multiple multinomial logistic regressions (base outcome: Postponed dental visits).

Author Contributions: Conceptualization, A.H., F.D.B. and H.-H.K.; formal analysis, A.H.; methodology, A.H.; supervision, H.-H.K.; writing—original draft, A.H.; Writing—review and editing, A.H., F.D.B., L.H., B.K. and H.-H.K. All authors have read and agreed to the published version of the manuscript.

Funding: This research was funded by DFG, grant number 3970/11-1; further funding via BZgA, RKI, ZPID, University of Erfurt (no funding numbers). The funders had no role in study design, data collection, interpretation, or the decision to submit the work for publication.

Institutional Review Board Statement: The study was conducted according to the guidelines of the Declaration of Helsinki, and approved by the Institutional Review Board of University of Erfurt (#202000302).

Informed Consent Statement: Informed consent was obtained from all individual participants included in the study.

Data Availability Statement: Data are not publicly available but interested parties may contact the authors for more information. The data are not publicly available due to ethical restrictions.

Acknowledgments: Germany's COVID-19 Snapshot Monitoring (COSMO) is a joint project of the University of Erfurt (Cornelia Betsch [PI], Lars Korn, Philipp Sprengholz, Philipp Schmid, Lisa Felgendreff, Sarah (RKI; Lothar H. Wieler, Patrick Schmich), the Federal Centre for Health Education (BZgA; Eitze), the Robert Koch Institute Heidrun Thaiss, Freia De Bock), the Leibniz

Centre for Psychological Information and Documentation (ZPID; Michael Bosnjak), the Science Media Center (SMC; Volker Stollorz), the Bernhard Nocht Institute for Tropical Medicine (BNITM; Michael Ramharter), and the Yale Institute for Global Health (Saad Omer).

Conflicts of Interest: The authors declare no conflict of interests.

References

1. Afonso-Souza, G.; Nadanovsky, P.; Chor, D.; Faerstein, E.; Werneck, G.; Lopes, C. Association between routine visits for dental checkup and self-perceived oral health in an adult population in Rio de Janeiro: The Pró-Saúde Study. *Community Dent. Oral Epidemiol.* **2007**, *35*, 393–400. [CrossRef] [PubMed]
2. Bottenberg, P.; Vanobbergen, J.; Declerck, D.; Carvalho, J.C. Oral health and healthcare utilization in Belgian dentate adults. *Community Dent. Oral Epidemiol.* **2019**, *47*, 381–388. [CrossRef] [PubMed]
3. Aarabi, G.; Valdez, R.; Spinler, K.; Walther, C.; Seedorf, U.; Heydecke, G.; König, H.-H.; Hajek, A. Determinants of Postponed Dental Visits Due to Costs: Evidence from the Survey of Health, Ageing, and Retirement in Germany. *Int. J. Environ. Res. Public Health* **2019**, *16*, 3344. [CrossRef] [PubMed]
4. Spinler, K.; Aarabi, G.; Walther, C.; Valdez, R.; Heydecke, G.; Buczak-Stec, E.; König, H.-H.; Hajek, A. Determinants of dental treatment avoidance: Findings from a nationally representative study. *Aging Clin. Exp. Res.* **2020**, 1–7. [CrossRef]
5. Kassebaum, N.; Bernabé, E.; Dahiya, M.; Bhandari, B.; Murray, C.; Marcenes, W. Global burden of severe tooth loss: A systematic review and meta-analysis. *J. Dent. Res.* **2014**, *93*, 20S–28S. [CrossRef]
6. Valdez, R.; Aarabi, G.; Spinler, K.; Walther, C.; Kofahl, C.; Buczak-Stec, E.; Heydecke, G.; König, H.-H.; Hajek, A. Do postponed dental visits for financial reasons reduce quality of life? Evidence from the Survey of Health, Ageing and Retirement in Europe. *Aging Clin. Exp. Res.* **2020**, 1–6. [CrossRef]
7. Müller, F.; Shimazaki, Y.; Kahabuka, F.; Schimmel, M. Oral health for an ageing population: The importance of a natural dentition in older adults. *Int. Dent. J.* **2017**, *67*, 7–13. [CrossRef]
8. Heyman, R.E.; Slep, A.; White-Ajmani, M.; Bulling, L.; Zickgraf, H.F.; Franklin, M.E.; Wolff, M.S. Dental fear and avoidance in treatment seekers at a large, urban dental clinic. *Oral Health Prev. Dent.* **2016**, *14*, 315–320.
9. Schwendicke, F.; Krois, J.; Gomez, J. Impact of SARS-CoV2 (Covid-19) on dental practices: Economic analysis. *J. Dent.* **2020**, *99*, 103387. [CrossRef]
10. Guo, H.; Zhou, Y.; Liu, X.; Tan, J. The impact of the COVID-19 epidemic on the utilization of emergency dental services. *J. Dent. Sci.* **2020**. [CrossRef]
11. Micheelis, W.; Süßlin, W. Einstellungen und Bewertungen der Bevölkerung zur zahnärztlichen Versorgung in Deutschland–Ergebnisse einer bundesweiten Umfrage. *Idz-Information* **2012**, *1*, 3–24.
12. Zok, K. Warten auf den Arzttermin. Ergebnisse einer Repräsentativumfrage unter GKV-und PKV-Versicherten. *WIdO-Monit.* **2007**, *4*, 1–7.
13. Passon, A.; Lüngen, M.; Gerber, A.; Redaelli, M.; Stock, S. Das Krankenversicherungssystem in Deutschland. *Gesundheitsökonomie* **2009**, 105–136. [CrossRef]
14. Betsch, C.; Wieler, L.H.; Habersaat, K. Monitoring behavioural insights related to COVID-19. *Lancet* **2020**, *395*, 1255–1256. [CrossRef]
15. Münnich, R.; Gabler, S. *2012: Stichprobenoptimierung und Schätzung in Zensus 2011*; Statistisches Bundesamt: Wiesbaden, Germany, 2012; Volume 21.
16. Betsch, C.; Wieler, L.; Bosnjak, M.; Ramharter, M.; Stollorz, V.; Omer, S. COVID-19 Snapshot MOnitoring (COSMO): Monitoring knowledge, risk perceptions, preventive behaviours, and public trust in the current coronavirus outbreak. *Psych. Arch.* **2020**. [CrossRef]
17. Hägglin, C.; Hakeberg, M.; Ahlqwist, M.; Sullivan, M.; Berggren, U. Factors associated with dental anxiety and attendance in middle-aged and elderly women. *Community Dent. Oral Epidemiol.* **2000**, *28*, 451–460. [CrossRef]
18. Watson, D.; Clark, L.A.; Carey, G. Positive and negative affectivity and their relation to anxiety and depressive disorders. *J. Abnorm. Psychol.* **1988**, *97*, 346. [CrossRef]
19. Boeira, G.; Correa, M.; Peres, K.; Peres, M.; Santos, I.; Matijasevich, A.; Barros, A.; Demarco, F. Caries is the main cause for dental pain in childhood: Findings from a birth cohort. *Caries Res.* **2012**, *46*, 488–495. [CrossRef]
20. Maciel, P.P.; Martelli Júnior, H.; Martelli, D.R.B.; Machado, R.A.; Andrade, P.V.d.; Perez, D.E.d.C.; Bonan, P.R.F. Covid-19 pandemic: Oral repercussions and its possible impact on oral health. *Pesqui. Bras. Odontopediatria Clin. Integr.* **2020**, *20*. [CrossRef]
21. Ren, Y.; Rasubala, L.; Malmstrom, H.; Eliav, E. Dental care and oral health under the clouds of COVID-19. *Jdr Clin. Transl. Res.* **2020**, 2380084420924385. [CrossRef]
22. Farook, F.F.; Nuzaim, M.N.M.; Ababneh, K.T.; Alshammari, A.; Alkadi, L. COVID-19 Pandemic: Oral Health Challenges and Recommendations. *Eur. J. Dent.* **2020**. [CrossRef]
23. Clarkson, J.E.; Pitts, N.B.; Goulao, B.; Boyers, D.; Ramsay, C.R.; Floate, R.; Braid, H.J.; Fee, P.A.; Ord, F.S.; Worthington, H.V.; et al. Risk-based, 6-monthly and 24-monthly dental check-ups for adults: The INTERVAL three-arm RCT. *Health Technol. Assess.* **2020**, *24*, 1–138. [CrossRef] [PubMed]

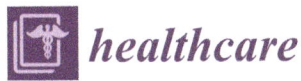

Article

Impact of the COVID-19 Pandemic on Manual Therapy Service Utilization within the Australian Private Healthcare Setting

Reidar P. Lystad [1,*], Benjamin T. Brown [2], Michael S. Swain [2] and Roger M. Engel [2]

[1] Australian Institute of Health Innovation, Macquarie University, Sydney 2109, Australia
[2] Department of Chiropractic, Macquarie University, Sydney 2109, Australia; benjamin.brown@mq.edu.au (B.T.B.); michael.swain@mq.edu.au (M.S.S.); roger.engel@mq.edu.au (R.M.E.)
* Correspondence: reidar.lystad@mq.edu.au

Received: 17 November 2020; Accepted: 11 December 2020; Published: 13 December 2020

Abstract: The COVID-19 pandemic has impacted a wide range of health services. This study aimed to quantify the impact of the COVID-19 pandemic on manual therapy service utilization within the Australian private healthcare setting during the first half of 2020. Quarterly data regarding the number and total cost of services provided were extracted for each manual therapy profession (i.e., chiropractic, osteopathy, and physiotherapy) for the period January 2015 to June 2020 from the Australian Prudential Regulation Authority. Time series forecasting methods were used to estimate absolute and relative differences between the forecasted and observed values of service utilization. An estimated 1.3 million (13.2%) fewer manual therapy services, with a total cost of AUD 84 million, were provided within the Australian private healthcare setting during the first half of 2020. Reduction in service utilization was considerably larger in the second quarter (21.7%) than in the first quarter (5.7%), and was larger in physiotherapy (20.6%) and osteopathy (12.7%) than in chiropractic (5.2%). The impact varied across states and territories, with the largest reductions in service utilization observed in New South Wales (17.5%), Australian Capital Territory (16.3%), and Victoria (16.2%). The COVID-19 pandemic has had a profound impact on manual therapy service utilization in Australia. The magnitude of the decline in service utilization varied considerably across professions and locations. The long-term consequences of this decline in manual therapy utilization remain to be determined.

Keywords: COVID-19; health services; cost; manual therapy; chiropractic; osteopathy; physiotherapy

1. Introduction

The novel coronavirus disease caused by severe acute respiratory syndrome coronavirus 2 (SARS-CoV-2) that emerged in Wuhan, China, in December 2019 (COVID-19) was declared a global pandemic by the World Health Organization on 11 March 2020 [1]. Major human events and natural calamities such as global pandemics have the potential to affect human behavior and access to resources, including healthcare seeking behavior and service utilization. There is emerging evidence that the COVID-19 pandemic has impacted a wide range of health services, including stroke emergency services [2–4], medical imaging services [5,6], and hospice care [7]. However, the impact of the COVID-19 pandemic on manual therapy service utilization is unknown.

In Australia, chiropractors, osteopaths, and physiotherapists are registered healthcare practitioners trained to diagnose, treat, and manage patients with musculoskeletal conditions. As of the first quarter of 2020, there were 5383 chiropractors, 2627 osteopaths, and 33,299 physiotherapists with general registration to practice in Australia [8–10]. The manual therapy services provided by these professions are predominately paid for by non-government sources (i.e., private health insurers and individuals).

Studies have documented increased utilization of manual therapy services over time in Australia, albeit with diverging trends across professions [11,12]. It has been estimated that approximately 21.6 million manual therapy services with a total cost of AUD 1.4 billion were provided within the Australian private healthcare setting annually in the period between 2013 and 2017, which represented a significant increase from the preceding five-year period [12]. It remains to be determined how these trends and figures have been impacted by the COVID-19 pandemic.

This study aimed to quantify the impact of the COVID-19 pandemic on manual therapy service utilization within the private healthcare setting in Australia. The specific objectives were to quantify the absolute and relative difference between forecasted and observed number and total cost of services during the first half of 2020 for each manual therapy profession.

2. Materials and Methods

2.1. Data Sources

Statistics on private health insurance industry activity in Australia are available from the Australian Prudential Regulation Authority (APRA) [13]. For the present study, we extracted quarterly data on the number and total cost of services for each manual therapy profession (i.e., chiropractic, osteopathy, and physiotherapy) from the first quarter (Q1) of 2015 to the second quarter (Q2) of 2020. We also extracted quarterly data on the estimated number of persons covered under private health insurance general treatment cover. A pyramid plot of the number of persons insured by sex and age group in 2020 Q2 is provided in Section A of the Supplementary Materials (Figure S1). Statistics on registered healthcare practitioners are available from the Australian Health Practitioner Regulation Agency (AHPRA) and each profession's registration board [8–10,14]. For this study, we extracted quarterly data on the number of registered providers from each manual therapy profession from 2015 Q1 to 2020 Q2. We did not include registrants listed as limited or non-practicing. We then estimated the number of providers working in the private sector for each profession as follows: For chiropractic and osteopathy, 100% of registrants were taken to be working in the private sector because neither of these professions contribute to service provision in the public sector. For physiotherapy, 63.5% of registrants were taken to be working in the private sector, as estimated by a National Health Workforce Report [15].

2.2. Operational Definitions

There are three types of private health insurance coverage in Australia: hospital treatment only, general treatment only, and combined hospital and general treatment. General treatment cover includes most services for preventing or managing injuries, diseases, and conditions that are provided outside of the hospital setting. However, it excludes services for chronic disease management that are covered by Medicare. A service was defined as one visit to a healthcare provider.

2.3. Data Management and Analysis

All dollar values were adjusted for inflation using the Reserve Bank of Australia's online inflation calculator and reported in second quarter of 2020 Australian dollars [16]. The main outcome variables were number of services per quarter and total cost of services per quarter. The number of providers was used as the denominator to calculate the following secondary outcome variables: number of services per provider per quarter and total cost per provider per quarter. The number of individuals with general treatment cover was used as the denominator to calculate the following secondary outcome variables: number of services per 100,000 insured population per quarter and total cost of services per 100,000 insured population per quarter.

Time series forecasting involved fitting seasonal autoregressive integrated moving average (ARIMA) models of service utilization data from 2015 to 2019 using the methods described by Hyndman and Athanasopoulos [17]. The seasonal ARIMA models provided estimates that account for seasonality and trends over time. Point forecast estimates with 95% prediction intervals for 2020 Q1 and Q2 were calculated from the seasonal ARIMA models and compared against observed values. The resulting mean errors and mean percentage errors were used as measures of absolute and relative impact. All statistical analyses were conducted using R, version 3.5.1 (R Foundation for Statistical Computing, Vienna, Austria) using the forecast and hts packages.

3. Results

For the three manual therapy professions combined, an estimated 1,322,370 (13.2%) fewer services were provided during the first half of 2020. The estimated reduction in total cost of services provided amounted to AUD 83,972,816 (11.5%). The combined estimated relative reduction in quarterly number and total cost of services provided was greater in Q2 (21.7% and 16.6%, respectively) than in Q1 (5.7% and 6.8%, respectively).

During the first half of 2020, the estimated relative reduction in number of services provided was considerably larger in physiotherapy (20.6%) and osteopathy (12.7%) than in chiropractic (5.2%). Figure 1 shows a time series plot of observed values and point forecast estimates with 95% prediction intervals of the quarterly number of services provided by each manual therapy profession from 2015 to 2020 Q2. Similarly, the estimated relative reduction in the quarterly total cost of services provided was considerably larger in physiotherapy (17.0%) and osteopathy (13.1%) than in chiropractic (4.7%). Figure 2 shows a time series plot of observed values and point forecast estimates with 95% prediction intervals of the quarterly total cost of services provided by each manual therapy profession from 2015 to 2020 Q2. Table 1 provides an overview of observed values, point forecast estimates, mean absolute error, and mean absolute percentage error of the quarterly number and total cost of services provided by each manual therapy profession during 2020 Q1 and Q2.

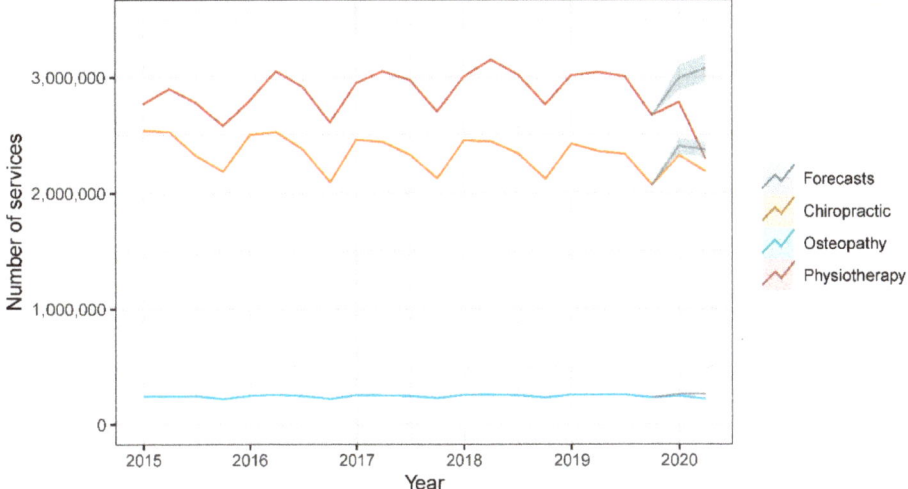

Figure 1. Time series plot of observed values and point forecast estimates with 95% prediction intervals of the quarterly number of services provided by each manual therapy profession from 2015 to 2020 Q2.

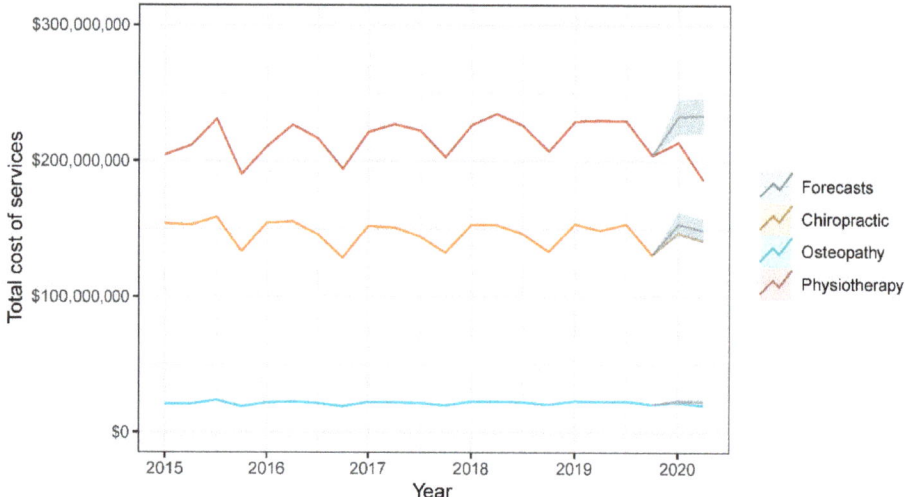

Figure 2. Time series plot of observed values and point forecast estimates with 95% prediction intervals of the quarterly total cost of services provided by each manual therapy profession from 2015 to 2020 Q2.

Table 1. Observed values, forecast point estimates, mean errors, and mean percentage errors of the quarterly number and total cost of services provided by each manual therapy profession in Australia during 2020 Q1 and Q2.

	Chiropractic	Osteopathy	Physiotherapy
2020 Q1			
Number of services			
Observed	2,321,874	246,011	2,783,058
Forecast point estimate	2,402,991	260,956	2,992,101
(95% prediction interval)	(2,332,444 to 2,473,537)	(253,739 to 268,173)	(2,880,914 to 3,103,288)
Mean error	−81,117	−14,945	−209,043
Mean percentage error	−3.5%	−6.1%	−7.5%
Total cost			
Observed	AUD 147,289,851	AUD 22,268,311	AUD 213,939,030
Forecast point estimate	AUD 153,756,465	AUD 23,253,647	AUD 232,693,899
(95% prediction interval)	(AUD 144,918,266 to 162,594,663)	(AUD 21,596,951 to 24,910,343)	(AUD 219,505,714 to 245,882,084)
Mean error	−AUD 6,466,613	−AUD 985,336	−AUD 18,754,869
Mean percentage error	−4.4%	−4.4%	−8.8%
2020 Q2			
Number of services			
Observed	2,183,321	217,595	2,289,773
Forecast point estimate	2,370,623	261,755	3,075,576
(95% prediction interval)	(2,300,077 to 2,441,170)	(254,538 to 268,972)	(2,954,135 to 3,197,016)
Mean error	−187,302	−44,160	−785,803
Mean percentage error	−8.6%	−20.3%	−34.3%
Total cost			
Observed	AUD 141,323,394	AUD 20,076,981	AUD 186,367,287
Forecast point estimate	AUD 149,092,929	AUD 22,939,482	AUD 233,501,248
(95% prediction interval)	(AUD 140,254,731 to 157,931,128)	(AUD 21,282,786 to 24,596,178)	AUD 220,313,063 to 246,689,433)
Mean error	−AUD 7,769,535	−AUD 2,862,502	−AUD 47,133,961
Mean percentage error	−5.5%	−14.3%	−25.3%

The estimated relative reduction in number and cost of services provided during the first half of 2020 varied by Australian state and territory. The estimated relative reduction in number of services provided was largest in New South Wales (17.5%), followed by Australian Capital Territory (16.3%), Victoria (16.2%), Tasmania (15.0%), South Australia (10.3%), Queensland (8.7%), Western Australia (7.9%), and Northern Territory (0.3%). Similarly, the estimated relative reduction in total cost of services provided was largest in New South Wales (15.6%) and Australian Capital Territory (15.6%), followed by Victoria (15.0%), Tasmania (11.2%), South Australia (9.3%), Western Australia (7.9%), Queensland (6.4%), and Northern Territory (0.9%). Figures 3 and 4 are heatmaps depicting the estimated mean percentage error in number and total cost of services, respectively, provided by the three manual therapy professions during the first half of 2020 across Australian states and territories.

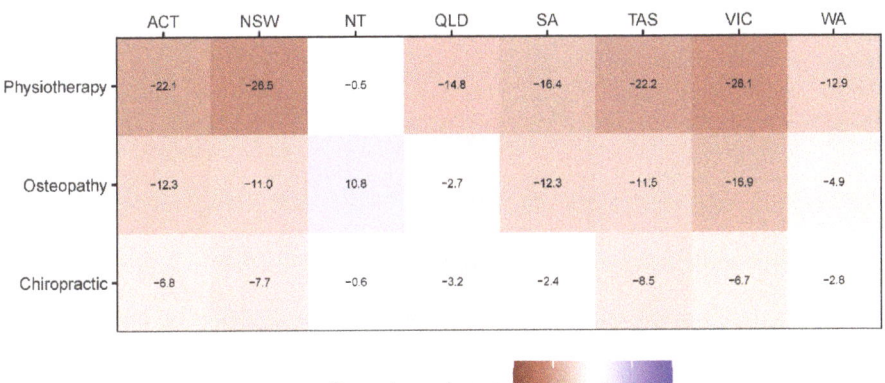

Figure 3. Heatmap of the estimated mean percentage error in number of services provided by each manual therapy profession during the first half of 2020 across Australian states and territories.

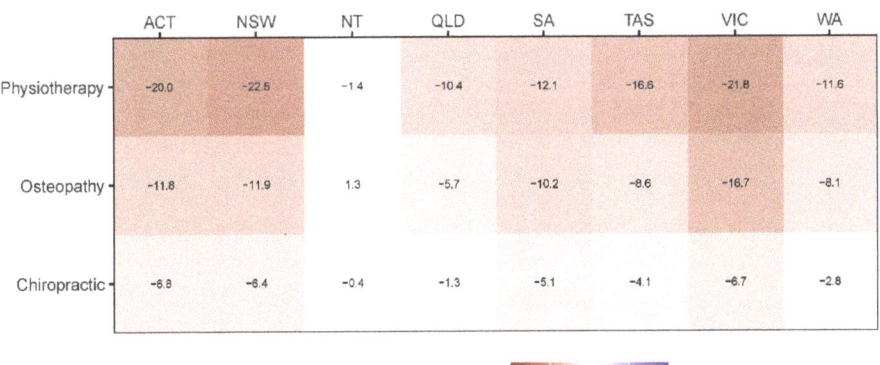

Figure 4. Heatmap of the estimated mean percentage error in total cost of services provided by each manual therapy profession during the first half of 2020 across Australian states and territories.

Because the number of individuals with general treatment cover and the number of manual therapy providers varied from quarter to quarter, supplementary analyses were conducted using secondary outcome variables and are presented in the Supplementary Materials (Sections B and C, respectively). These supplementary analyses generated similar estimates of the percentage change in manual therapy service utilization.

4. Discussion

This is the first study to estimate the impact of the COVID-19 pandemic on manual therapy service utilization. During the first half of 2020, the COVID-19 pandemic coincided with approximately 1.3 million fewer chiropractic, osteopathy, and physiotherapy services provided within the Australian private healthcare system. The associated loss of revenue was estimated to be AUD 84 million. Physiotherapy incurred the largest relative reduction in service provision and revenue, while chiropractic was found to be the least impacted of the three manual therapy professions. Geographically, the largest relative reductions in manual therapy service utilization were observed in the south-eastern corner of mainland Australia (i.e., New South Wales, Australian Capital Territory, and Victoria).

Our findings show that the COVID-19 pandemic has had a profound impact on manual therapy service utilization in Australia. It is not unexpected to observe disruption of health services during a global pandemic. While much of the initial disruption of health services has been characterized by the surge in demand for front-line care of COVID-19 patients, there has also been a concomitant reduction in or discontinuation of prevention and rehabilitation services for noncommunicable diseases. For instance, the World Health Organization reported that more than half of the countries surveyed had partially or completely disrupted services for the treatment or clinical management of hypertension, diabetes and diabetes-related complications, cancer, and cardiovascular emergencies [18]. A similar situation exists in Australia, where there have been marked reductions in a wide range of health services, including breast and prostate cancer screenings [19,20], pediatric orthopedic hospital services [21], trauma care in Emergency Departments [22,23], and initiation of cardiopulmonary resuscitation by Emergency Medical Services in public areas [24]. It is important to note that our findings encompass only the initial disruption caused by the COVID-19 pandemic. It remains to be determined whether the decline in manual therapy service utilization persists beyond the first half of 2020, whether manual therapy service utilization returns to pre-pandemic levels after the virus has been eliminated, and whether economic factors such as sustained or transient changes in disposable income, uptake of private health insurance, and cost of services have any lasting effects on healthcare-seeking behavior and manual therapy service utilization. Future studies are encouraged to explore these unresolved questions.

The magnitude of the decline in manual therapy service utilization during the COVID-19 pandemic was not uniform across the three professions, with physiotherapy and chiropractic experiencing the largest and smallest relative reductions, respectively. The exact reason for this difference is unclear, but it may be related to differences in revenue streams (e.g., proportion derived from private health insurance) and patient characteristics (e.g., level of disposable income) across the three professions [12]. For instance, as the COVID-19 pandemic has unfolded and loss of income became more prevalent in the population, perhaps Australians have forfeited their private health insurance with general treatment cover as a cost-saving measure. While this explanation may sound reasonable given the circumstances, it does not explain why there was a larger decline in physiotherapy service utilization relative to chiropractic and osteopathy. Nor does it explain the fact that the results from our supplementary analyses of service utilization per 100,000 insured persons were very similar to our main findings, which suggests that any changes in the number of insured persons are unlikely to explain the observed differences. An alternative explanation may be differences in case-mix across the three manual therapy professions. Although this explanation is not supported by the scope of practice of the three professions, which all state that they diagnose and treat musculoskeletal conditions, industry reports indicate that physiotherapy provides more specialized services (e.g., neurological rehabilitation, geriatric services, and sports injury prevention and rehabilitation) than osteopathy and chiropractic [25,26]. Thus, it is conceivable that public health orders and social restrictions related to the COVID-19 pandemic (e.g., stay-at-home directives, limited access to aged care facilities, and shutdown of community sport activities) may have resulted in a marked reduction in utilization of specialist physiotherapy services. Although this may explain the larger relative reduction in physiotherapy service utilization (20.6%), it does not adequately explain the differences in relative reduction in services between osteopathy (12.7%) and chiropractic (5.2%). Further research is needed to examine the factors influencing healthcare-seeking behavior and manual therapy service utilization during the COVID-19 pandemic and to elucidate the underlying reasons for the observed differences across the three manual therapy professions.

There are strengths and limitations of the present study. This research builds on our previous reports of manual therapy service utilization within the Australian private healthcare setting [11,12]. We added an inflation adjustment for all dollar values to remove the effect of inflation from our analyses. More importantly, we applied sophisticated analytical techniques to produce forecasts that account for both seasonal variation and long-term trends across professions and geographical regions (i.e., states and territories). In an attempt to account for changes in the number of providers and people with private health insurance, we provided supplementary analyses using secondary outcome variables (i.e., number and total cost of services provided per provider and per 100,000 persons with private health insurance). These supplementary analyses produced very similar estimates of the impact of the COVID-19 pandemic on manual therapy service utilization. Lastly, because our study was limited to private health insurance data, the estimates presented herein can only be generalized to services provided under private health insurance general treatment cover.

5. Conclusions

The COVID-19 pandemic has had a profound impact on manual therapy service utilization in Australia. The magnitude of the decline in service utilization varied considerably across professions and locations. The long-term consequences of this decline in manual therapy utilization remains to be determined.

Supplementary Materials: The following are available online at http://www.mdpi.com/2227-9032/8/4/558/s1, Section A: Figure S1: Pyramid plot depicting the number of persons insured under general treatment cover by sex and age group in the second quarter of 2020; Section B: Figure S2: Time series plot of observed values and point forecast estimates with 95% prediction intervals of the quarterly number of services provided per 100,000 insured persons by each manual therapy profession from 2015 to 2020 Q2; Figure S3: Time series plot of observed values and point forecast estimates with 95% prediction intervals of the quarterly total cost of services provided per 100,000 insured persons by each manual therapy profession from 2015 to 2020 Q2; Table S1: Observed values, forecast point estimates with 95% prediction intervals, mean errors, and mean percentage errors of the quarterly number and total cost of services provided per 100,000 insured persons by each manual therapy profession in Australia during 2020 Q1 and Q2; Figure S4: Heatmap of the estimated mean percentage error in number of services provided per 100,000 insured persons by each manual therapy profession during the first half of 2020 across Australian states and territories; Figure S5: Heatmap of the estimated mean percentage error in total cost of services provided per 100,000 insured persons by each manual therapy profession during the first half of 2020 across Australian states and territories; Section C: Figure S6: Time series plot of observed values and point forecast estimates with 95% prediction intervals of the quarterly number of services provided per provider by each manual therapy profession from 2015 to 2020 Q2; Figure S7: Time series plot of observed values and point forecast estimates with 95% prediction intervals of the quarterly total cost of services provided per provider by each manual therapy profession from 2015 to 2020 Q2; Table S2: Observed values, forecast point estimates with 95% prediction intervals, mean errors, and mean percentage errors of the quarterly number and total cost of services provided per provider by each manual therapy profession in Australia during 2020 Q1 and Q2; Figure S8: Heatmap of the estimated mean percentage error in number of services provided per provider by each manual therapy profession during the first half of 2020 across Australian states and territories; Figure S9: Heatmap of the estimated mean percentage error in total cost of services provided per provider by each manual therapy profession during the first half of 2020 across Australian states and territories.

Author Contributions: Conceptualization, R.P.L., B.T.B., M.S.S., and R.M.E.; methodology, R.P.L., B.T.B., M.S.S., and R.M.E.; formal analysis, R.P.L.; writing—original draft preparation, R.P.L., B.T.B., and M.S.S.; writing—review and editing, R.P.L., B.T.B., M.S.S., and R.M.E.; visualization, R.P.L. All authors have read and agreed to the published version of the manuscript.

Funding: This research received no external funding.

Conflicts of Interest: The authors declare no conflict of interest.

References

1. World Health Organization. WHO Director-General's Opening Remarks at the Media Briefing on COVID-19—11 March 2020. Available online: https://www.who.int/dg/speeches/detail/who-director-general-s-opening-remarks-at-the-media-briefing-on-covid-19---11-march-2020 (accessed on 23 July 2020).
2. Desai, S.M.; Guyette, F.X.; Martin-Gill, C.; Jadhav, A.P. Collateral damage—Impact of a pandemic on stroke emergency services. *J. Stroke Cerebrovasc. Dis.* **2020**, *29*, 104988. [CrossRef] [PubMed]
3. Kristoffersen, E.S.; Jahr, S.H.; Thommessen, B.; Rønning, O.M. Effect of COVID-19 pandemic on stroke admission rates in a Norwegian population. *Acta Neurol. Scand.* **2020**, *142*, 632–636. [CrossRef] [PubMed]
4. Bersano, A.; Kraemer, M.; Touzé, E.; Weber, R.; Alamowitch, S.; Sibon, I.; Pantoni, L. Stroke care during the COVID-19 pandemic: Experience from three large European countries. *Eur. J. Neurol.* **2020**, *27*, 1794–1800. [CrossRef] [PubMed]
5. Parikh, K.D.; Ramaiya, N.H.; Kikano, E.G.; Tirumani, S.H.; Pandya, H.; Stovicek, B.; Sunshine, J.L.; Plecha, D.M. COVID-19 Pandemic impact on decreased imaging utilization: A single institutional experience. *Acad. Radiol.* **2020**, *27*, 1204–1213. [CrossRef] [PubMed]
6. Duszak, R.; Maze, J.; Sessa, C.; Fleishon, H.B.; Golding, L.P.; Nicola, G.N.; Hughes, D.R. Characteristics of coronavirus disease 2019 (COVID-19) community practice declines in noninvasive diagnostic imaging professional work. *J. Am. Coll. Radiol.* **2020**, *17*, 1453–1459. [CrossRef] [PubMed]
7. Chou, Y.-C.; Yen, Y.-F.; Feng, R.-C.; Wu, M.-P.; Lee, Y.-L.; Chu, D.; Huang, S.-J.; Curtis, J.R.; Hu, H.-Y. Impact of the COVID-19 pandemic on the utilization of hospice care services: A cohort study in Taiwan. *J. Pain Symptom Manag.* **2020**, *60*, e1–e6. [CrossRef] [PubMed]
8. Chiropractic Board of Australia. Statistics. Available online: https://www.chiropracticboard.gov.au/About-the-Board/Statistics.aspx (accessed on 23 July 2020).
9. Osteopathy Board of Australia. Statistics. Available online: https://www.osteopathyboard.gov.au/About/Statistics.aspx (accessed on 23 July 2020).
10. Physiotherapy Board of Australia. Statistics. Available online: http://www.physiotherapyboard.gov.au/about/statistics.aspx (accessed on 23 July 2020).
11. Engel, R.M.; Brown, B.T.; Swain, M.S.; Lystad, R.P. The provision of chiropractic, physiotherapy and osteopathic services within the Australian private health-care system: A report of recent trends. *Chiropr. Man. Therap.* **2014**, *22*, 3. [CrossRef] [PubMed]
12. Lystad, R.P.; Brown, B.T.; Swain, M.S.; Engel, R.M. Service utilisation trends in the manual therapy professions within the Australian private healthcare setting between 2008 and 2017. *Chiropr. Man. Therap.* **2020**, *28*, 49. [CrossRef] [PubMed]
13. Australian Prudential Regulation Authority. Available online: https://www.apra.gov.au/ (accessed on 23 July 2020).
14. Australian Health Practitioner Regulation Agency. Available online: https://www.ahpra.gov.au/ (accessed on 23 July 2020).
15. Australian Institute of Health and Welfare. *Allied Health Work Force 2012*; Australian Institute of Health and Welfare: Canberra, Australia, 2013.
16. Reserve Bank of Australia. Inflation Calculator. Available online: https://www.rba.gov.au/calculator/ (accessed on 14 October 2020).
17. Hyndman, R.J.; Athanasopoulos, G. *Forecasting: Principles and Practice*, 3rd ed.; OTexts: Melbourne, Australia, 2018.
18. World Health Organization. COVID-19 Significantly Impacts Health Services for Noncommunicable Diseases. Available online: https://www.who.int/news/item/01-06-2020-covid-19-significantly-impacts-health-services-for-noncommunicable-diseases (accessed on 6 November 2020).
19. Cancer Australia. *Review of the Impact of COVID-19 on Medical Services and Procedures in Australia Utilising MBS Data: Skin, Breast and Colorectal Cancers, and Telehealth Services*; Cancer Australia: Sydney, Australia, 2020.
20. Australian Institute of Health and Welfare. Cancer Screening and COVD-19 in Australia. Available online: https://www.aihw.gov.au/reports/cancer-screening/cancer-screening-and-covid-19-in-australia/contents/how-has-covid-19-affected-australias-cancer-screening-programs (accessed on 6 November 2020).

21. Wong, F.L.; Antoniou, G.; Williams, N.; Cundy, P.J. Disruption of paediatric orthopaedic hospital services due to the COVID-19 pandemic in a region with minimal COVID-19 illness. *J. Child. Orthop.* **2020**, *14*, 245–251. [CrossRef] [PubMed]
22. Harris, D.; Ellis, D.Y.; Gorman, D.; Foo, N.; Haustead, D. Impact of COVID-19 social restrictions on trauma presentations in South Australia. *Emerg. Med. Australas.* **2020**. [CrossRef]
23. Probert, A.C.; Sivakumar, B.S.; An, V.; Nicholls, S.L.; Shatrov, J.G.; Symes, M.J.; Ellis, A.M. Impact of COVID-19-related social restrictions on orthopaedic trauma in a level 1 trauma centre in Sydney: The first wave. *ANZ J. Surg.* **2020**. [CrossRef]
24. Ball, J.; Nehme, Z.; Bernard, S.; Stub, D.; Stephenson, M.; Smith, K. Collateral damage: Hidden impact of the COVID-19 pandemic on the out-of-hospital cardiac arrest system-of-care. *Resuscitation* **2020**, *156*, 157–163. [CrossRef] [PubMed]
25. Richardson, A. *Chiropractic and Osteopathic Services in Australia. Industry Report Q8534*; IBISWorld: Melbourne, Australia, 2019.
26. Richardson, A. *Physiotherapy Services in Australia. Industry Report Q8533*; IBISWorld: Melbourne, Australia, 2019.

Publisher's Note: MDPI stays neutral with regard to jurisdictional claims in published maps and institutional affiliations.

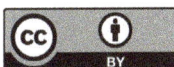

© 2020 by the authors. Licensee MDPI, Basel, Switzerland. This article is an open access article distributed under the terms and conditions of the Creative Commons Attribution (CC BY) license (http://creativecommons.org/licenses/by/4.0/).

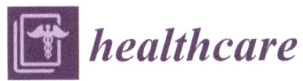

Article

COVID-19 and Psychological Health of Female Saudi Arabian Population: A Cross-Sectional Study

Syed Mohammed Basheeruddin Asdaq [1,*], Sara Abdulrahman Alajlan [1], Yahya Mohzari [2], Mohammed Asad [3], Ahmad Alamer [4,5], Ahmed A. Alrashed [6], Naira Nayeem [7] and Sreeharsha Nagaraja [8,9]

1. College of Pharmacy, AlMaarefa University, Riyadh 13713, Saudi Arabia; emadfaiqa@gmail.com
2. Pharmacy Department, Clinical Pharmacy Section, King Saud Medical City, Riyadh 12746, Saudi Arabia; yali2016@hotmail.com
3. Department of Clinical Laboratory Science, College of Applied Medical Sciences, Shaqra University, Shaqra 11911, Saudi Arabia; basheer_1@rediffmail.com
4. Department of Pharmacy Practice and Science, College of Pharmacy, University of Arizona, Tucson, AZ 85721, USA; mhospital1920@gmail.com
5. Department of Clinical Pharmacy, Prince Sattam Bin Abdulaziz University, Alkharj 11942, Saudi Arabia
6. Pharmaceutical Service Department, Main Hospital, King Fahad Medical City, Riyadh 11564, Saudi Arabia; alarashed@gmail.com
7. Department of Pharmaceutical Chemistry, Northern Border University, Arar 73214, Saudi Arabia; farhana.basheer13@gmail.com
8. Department of Pharmaceutical Sciences, College of Clinical Pharmacy, King Faisal University, Al-Ahsa 31982, Saudi Arabia; sharsha@kfu.edu.sa
9. Department of Pharmaceutics, Vidya Siri College of Pharmacy, Off Sarjapura Road, Bengaluru 560 035, Karnataka, India
* Correspondence: sasdaq@mcst.edu.sa; Tel.: +966-1-403555-3399

Received: 17 November 2020; Accepted: 5 December 2020; Published: 9 December 2020

Abstract: The influence of the COVID-19 pandemic is unprecedented on physical and mental health. This study aimed to determine the impact of the COVID-19 event on mental health among Saudi Arabian females of Riyadh by a cross-sectional study design. The samples of the study were recruited using convenience and snowball sampling methods. The questionnaire is composed of items related to sociodemographic profile, general mental status, negative attitude scale, impact of event (COVID-19 pandemic) scale (R) and negative health impact. The data obtained were analyzed using multivariate regression analysis. Out of the 797 samples (34.58 ± 12.89 years), 457 (57.34%) belonged to an age group of ≥25 years. The average BMI of the participants was 26.73 (kg/m^2). Significantly ($p = 0.000$), a large proportion of the participants were overweight and unemployed. Age group (>25 years) have more odds for abnormal mental status (OR; 1.592), development of negative attitudes (OR; 1.986), the intense impact of COVID-19 events (OR; 1.444) and susceptibility to attain negative health impacts (OR; 1.574). High body weight is another risk factor for altered mental status, negative attitude and developing impact of COVID-19 quickly. Overall, the COVID-19 pandemic was directly associated with stress (53%), anxiety (63%) and depression (44%) in our sample population. There is an urgent need for psychological counseling for the distressed population.

Keywords: COVID-19; mental health; Impact of event scale; negative attitude; Saudi Arabian females

1. Introduction

The unprecedented situation of COVID-19 presents a remarkable threat to the health of the general public. The presence of this highly contagious disease with the unpredictable extent of morbidity and mortality rates has an impact on almost all aspects of daily life [1]. During this difficult pandemic time, it is likely that mental health issues may get exacerbated due to perceive fear, worry, and stress because of uncertainty or factors over which humans have no control. More than one-third of the adults from the United States have shown symptoms of anxiety or depression during the pandemic, in contrast, to a figure of one in ten; from January to June 2019 [2]. In addition to the threat of getting infected with the virus, alterations in daily activities like restricted movements and strict maintenance of social distancing in several countries, new normal of work from home, partial or complete loss of a job, virtual classes for children, and avoidance of contact with friends and relatives, are considered as major contributors for altered mental functions during this crisis [3]. Concerning the susceptibility for psychological disturbance, the impact of a major epidemic is directly associated with the ability of a person to cope up with the situation. It is not wrong to say that almost the entire population has experienced some degree of mental distress during this difficult time, but the significant impact is seen only in vulnerable individuals. Particularly those people who got infected with the disease, those at high risk, such as the geriatric population, immunocompromised individuals, those living or receiving care in congregate settings, and people with preexisting psychiatric or substance abuse problems, possess an enhanced risk for abnormal psychosocial outcomes [4]. On top of that, long-term lockdown due to pandemic also results in limited access to healthcare that invariably results in mental health issues [5]. Moreover, females are more likely to develop psychological burden than males [6]. Additionally, a significant impact on mental health is also reported in people who have limited resources to use virtual social and health awareness services [7]. In addition, it is necessary to understand that all psychological illness and socialization issues are not necessarily can be termed as diseases; most of them temporary reactions to abnormal situations. However, it must be addressed in time to prevent the occurrence of its consequences.

Recently published articles emphatically describe the implication of COVID-19 on the mental health of health care professionals [8] as they are the front line warriors for this virus, and also several reports published on the implication of this situation on the educational system [9]. The reports describing the role of the pandemic on the mental status of the community [8,10] are also published elsewhere. However, there is a scarcity of data on the direct impact of COVID-19 on the mental status of the female population of Saudi Arabia. Hence, this study aimed to determine the impact of the COVID-19 event on mental health and its related lifestyle habits among Saudi Arabian females of Riyadh.

2. Materials and Methods

2.1. Sampling

This is a cross-sectional study carried out from March 2020 until the end of August 2020. The study period coincides with the progression of COVID-19 cases in Saudi Arabia. The number of new cases has been increasing many-fold, ranging from 100 odd cases in March 2020 up to 4919 cases on 17 July 2020. The number of deaths was in single digits during March that went to a peak of 58 deaths on 5 July 2020. However, due to stringent regulations of Saudi Arabian authorities, the spread of the pandemic was well controlled, with the number of new recoveries per day was almost similar to or higher than new reported COVID-19 cases. Additionally, the media of Saudi Arabia was helping the governmental authorities in restricting the spread of rumors. Overall, the situation was alarming but well under control. Ethical approval to conduct this study was obtained from the Research Committee of College of Pharmacy, AlMaarefa University, Riyadh, with approval number (MCST (AU)-COP 2001/RC). Only female adults (aged ≥ 18 years) of Saudi Arabian nationality who provided verbal informed consent and reside in Riyadh (Saudi Arabia) were recruited in the study using convenience and snowball sampling methods. The content validity and reliability check of the questionnaire were done by Cronbach's alpha. The validated questionnaire was translated into the Arabic language, and linguistic validation was done to validate the conceptual translation of the questionnaire with the help of two qualified bilingual (English and Arabic languages) health science researchers. Pretest of the

Arabic version of the questionnaire was conducted to assess the clarity of the questionnaire, suitability to the participants, the time required to complete the questionnaire and to know the possible obstacles.

The sample size was calculated (http://sampsize.sourceforge.net) based on the 28% prevalence of psychological illness in the female population of Saudi Arabia reported in one of the studies [11] with a 5% as a precision percentage and a 95% confidence level. The required sample size was 310 for the infinite population.

2.2. Study Questionnaire

The questionnaire used in this study had five major sections: (1) sociodemographic information such as age, education level, employment status, height and weight (to calculate BMI); (2) General mental status; (3) Negative attitude scale; (4) Impact of event (COVID-19 pandemic) Scale (R) and (5) Negative health impact.

2.3. General Mental Status (GMH)

The validated Arabic version of the 8-item section with Cronbach's alpha of 0.70 was used to explore the basic mental profile of the participants during this pandemic. The items included were perceived depression status during the pandemic, medication used to control psychological burden, soliciting psychologist help, participation in mental health program during the pandemic, joining audio broadcast of mental health issues, initiating stress reliever exercise, nightmares during the pandemic and developing bad habits. The response for each question was scored 0 (no) and 1 (yes). A cutoff of ≥3 was used to reflect abnormal mental status.

2.4. Negative Attitude Scale (NA)

There were seven questions included in this section that were focused on elucidating the perceived negative attitude developed during the pandemic. These questions had a Cronbach's alpha of 0.92. The questions were meant to evaluate the interest level, social life, feelings of frustration and despair, tension level, ability to focus and mood status. The responses for each question were scored 0 (never), 1 (rare), 2 (sometimes), 3 (most of the time) and 4 (always), with a lower score indicating a low negative attitude. A cutoff of ≥ 8 was used to reflect the presence of a negative attitude.

2.5. Impact of Event (COVID-19 Pandemic) Scale (R) (IES)

Daniel Weiss and Charles Marmar developed the first draft of the impact of event scale (IES) in 1997 [12] to parallel the DSM-IV criteria, subscale with hyperarousal items were included into IES and renamed as IES-R [13]. This scale comprises of total 22 items measured on a 5-point Likert scale rated from 0 to 4 (0 = not at all, 1 = a little, 2 = moderately, 3 = quite a bit and 4 = extremely) based on the extent to which 22 items described in the scale has caused distress to the participants in the last 7 days with reference to COVID-19. The consistency of the items was found to have Cronbach's alpha of 0.94. The cutoff score reported in earlier literature ranges from 25 to 40, with a score of more than cutoff indicate a person at high risk for psychological problems [14]. Since this study was done during the time of the event, the investigators decided on a mean score of 35 as the cutoff point to validate the impact of COVID-19 in the participants. Intrusion (items 1, 2, 3, 6, 9, 14, 16 and 20), avoidance (items 5, 7, 8, 11, 12, 13, 17 and 22) and hyperarousal (items 4, 10, 15, 18, 19, 21) are three subscales to this questionnaire.

2.6. Negative Mental Health Impact (NHI)

Participants were asked to share their opinion on the six validated questions about negative mental health impacts of the pandemic compared to the pre-pandemic period; these questions had a Cronbach's alpha of 0.88 [15]. The stress of work, financial burden, stress from home, fear due to the COVID-19 pandemic, apprehension due to the COVID-19 pandemic, and helpless feelings due to the

COVID-19 pandemic were tested in this section. The categorical responses recorded were either yes (score 0) or no (Score 1). A total score of ≥3 was termed as the cutoff score for considering the presence of negative health impact due to pandemic.

2.7. Statistical Analysis

The data collected was entered into SPSS IBM statistical package (version 25, IBM, Armonk, NY, USA). All results of quantitative variables were reported either as mean or frequency (percentage) (%). A chi-squared test was employed to assess if there was a significant association between categorical variables. Risk estimates of the sociodemographic factors (age, educational level and BMI) on GMH, NA, IES and NHI were determined and expressed as an odds ratio. Finally, multivariate linear regression analysis was done to assess the difference in dependent and independent variables, including age, educational level, and body weight (BMI). A *p*-value of less than 0.05 was considered significant.

3. Results

3.1. Characteristics of the Participants

Of the 1191 responses received for our questionnaire, 216 responses were excluded from our study due to incomplete information on the sociodemographic profile. Out of the remaining 797 samples (average age 34.58 years), 457 (57.34%) belonged to an age group of >25 years, and 340 (42.65%) were from the 18–25 years age group. Only 30% of the respondents were secondary school qualified, while the majority of them are better educated (69%). Most of the participants (64%) of this study were non-employed or students, whereas 36% of them were working. Concerning the status of body weight, a higher proportion of the included samples were overweight (66%), with only 34% representing normal weight. The average BMI of the participants was 26.73 (kg/m^2). Significantly ($p = 0.000$), a high percentage of the surveyors in the higher age group were overweight and unemployed (Table 1).

Table 1. Sociodemographic characteristics of the participants.

Variables	All, n (%)	18–25 Years, n (%)	>25 Years, n (%)	*p* Value [1]
Education level				
Higher qualification, n (%)	556 (69.8)	228 (67.1)	328 (71.8)	0.152
Secondary school, n (%)	241 (30.2)	112 (32.9)	129 (28.2)	
Employment status				
Employed, n (%)	287 (36)	93 (27.4)	194 (42.5)	0.000
Non employed, n (%)	371 (46.5)	113 (33.2)	258 (56.5)	
Students, n (%)	139 (17.4)	134 (39.4)	5 (1.1)	
BMI				
Normal weight, n (%)	273 (34.3)	158 (46.5)	115 (25.2)	0.000
Overweight, n (%)	524 (65.7)	182 (53.5)	342 (74.8)	

[1] Pearson chi-squared test.

3.2. General Mental Status, Negative Attitude, IES, Negative Health Impact by Age

The overall mean general mental status score of 1.5 ± 0.059 (mean ± SEM) was noted among the participants with a significantly ($p = 0.001$) high level of abnormal mental status in a higher age group (Odds ratio, 1.304) compared to lower to age group (Table 2). The average score for negative attitude was 7.79 ± 0.239, with a risk estimate of 1.304 for the higher age group. There was no association of age on the impact of event scale (IES on COVID-19) with an overall average of 20.83 ± 0.569 among the participants. However, the age group of ≥25 years had a relatively bigger risk estimate (1.249) for the IES score. Additionally, a significant ($p = 0.001$) link was found between negative health impact and age of the participants, with an overall mean score of 2.41 ± 0.062. The overall average of IES sub-scale intrusion, avoidance and hyperarousal were 7.55 ± 0.21, 7.05 ± 0.22 and 6.22 ± 0.5, respectively.

Table 2. General mental status, negative attitude, impact of event scale (IES), negative health impact by age.

Variables	All, n (%)	18–25 Years, n (%)	>25 Years, n (%)	p Value [1]
\multicolumn{5}{c}{General mental status}				
Normal, n (%)	614 (77)	372 (81.4)	242 (71.2)	
Abnormal, n (%)	183 (23)	85 (18.6)	98 (28.8)	0.001
Odds ratio (risk estimate) [2]		0.736	1.304	
\multicolumn{5}{c}{Negative attitude}				
Absent, n (%)	466 (58.5)	164 (48.2)	302 (66.1)	
Present, n (%)	331 (41.5)	176 (51.8)	155 (33.9)	0.000
Odds ratio (risk estimate) [2]		0.662	1.304	
\multicolumn{5}{c}{Impact of COVID-19 event}				
Absent, n (%)	640 (80.3)	258 (75.9)	382 (83.6)	
Present, n (%)	157 (19.7)	82 (24.1)	75 (16.4)	0.007
Odds ratio (risk estimate) [2]		0.772	1.249	
\multicolumn{5}{c}{Negative health impact}				
Absent, n (%)	446 (56)	167 (49.1)	279 (61.1)	
Present, n (%)	351 (44)	173 (50.9)	178 (38.9)	0.001
Odds ratio (risk estimate) [2]		0.760	1.234	

[1] Pearson chi-squared test; [2] risk estimate for 2 × 2 table.

3.3. General Mental Status, Negative Attitude, IES, Negative Health Impact by BMI

As shown in Table 3, overweight participants of this study had significantly abnormal mental status ($p = 0.000$), higher negative attitude ($p = 0.001$) and increase in the IES score (impact of COVID-19 event) ($p = 0.000$). However, there was no significant association between negative health impact and bodyweight. Similarly, overweight subjects of this study have shown a relatively higher risk for abnormal mental status (1.279), negative attitude (1.189), the impact of COVID-19 (1.249) and negative health impact (1.096).

Table 3. General mental status, negative attitude, IES, negative health impact by body weight (BMI).

Variables	All, n (%)	Normal Weight, n (%)	Overweight, n (%)	p Value [1]
\multicolumn{5}{c}{General mental status}				
Normal, n (%)	614 (77)	189 (69.2)	425 (81.1)	
Abnormal, n (%)	183 (23)	84 (30.8)	99 (18.9)	0.000
Odds ratio (risk estimate) [2]		0.671	1.279	
\multicolumn{5}{c}{Negative attitude}				
Absent, n (%)	466 (58.5)	138 (50.5)	328 (62.6)	
Present, n (%)	331 (41.5)	135 (49.5)	196 (37.4)	0.001
Odds ratio (risk estimate) [2]		0.726	1.189	
\multicolumn{5}{c}{Impact of COVID-19 event}				
Absent, n (%)	640 (80.3)	202 (74)	438 (83.6)	
Present, n (%)	157 (19.7)	71 (26)	86 (16.4)	0.001
Odds ratio (risk estimate) [2]		0.698	1.249	
\multicolumn{5}{c}{Negative health impact}				
Absent, n (%)	446 (56)	141 (51.6)	305 (58.2)	
Present, n (%)	351 (44)	132 (48.4)	219 (41.8)	0.077
Odds ratio (risk estimate) [2]		0.841	1.096	

[1] Pearson chi-squared test; [2] risk estimate for 2 × 2 table.

3.4. General Mental Status, Negative Attitude, IES, Negative Health Impact by Educational Level

There was no significant association noted when we compared education level with changes in the general mental status, development of negative attitude due to COVID, the impact of the COVID-19 on their general lifestyle and overall negative impact. On the contrary, participants with low educational level had a comparatively higher risk estimate for abnormal mental status (1.057), negative attitude (1.171) and negative health impact (1.019) (Table 4).

Table 4. General mental status, negative attitude, IES, negative health impact by educational level.

Variables	All, n (%)	Higher Qualification, n (%)	Secondary School, n (%)	p Value [1]
		General mental status		
Normal, n (%)	614 (77)	426 (76.6)	188 (78)	
Abnormal, n (%)	183 (23)	130 (23.4)	53 (22)	0.668
Odds ratio (risk estimate) [2]		0.977	1.057	
		Negative attitude		
Absent, n (%)	466 (58.5)	316 (56.8)	150 (62.2)	
Present, n (%)	331 (41.5)	240 (43.2)	91 (37.8)	0.155
Odds ratio (risk estimate) [2]		0.935	1.171	
		Impact of COVID-19 event		
Absent, n (%)	640 (80.3)	449 (80.8)	191 (79.3)	
Present, n (%)	157 (19.7)	107 (19.2)	50 (20.7)	0.624
Odds ratio (risk estimate) [2]		1.029	0.937	
		Negative health impact		
Absent, n (%)	446 (56)	310 (55.8)	136 (56.4)	
Present, n (%)	351 (44)	246 (44.2)	105 (43.6)	0.860
Odds ratio (risk estimate) [2]		0.92	1.019	

[1] Pearson chi-squared test; [2] risk estimate for 2 × 2 table.

Table 5. Multiple linear regression analysis.

Scale	Variable	B	Std. Error	Beta	p Value
General Mental status	Constant	1.224	0.194		0.000 *
	Age	0.465	0.175	1.592	0.008 *
	Educational level	−0.080	0.189	0.923	0.672
	BMI	−0.540	0.177	0.583	0.002 *
Negative attitude	Constant	0.252	0.167		0.132
	Age	0.686	0.151	1.986	0.000 *
	Educational level	−0.253	0.162	0.777	0.120
	BMI	−0.331	0.156	0.718	0.034 *
Impact of COVID-19 event	Constant	1.330	0.201		0.000 *
	Age	0.367	0.185	1.444	0.047 *
	Educational level	0.103	0.195	1.108	0.599
	BMI	−0.505	0.187	0.603	0.007 *
Negative health impact	Constant	0.068	0.164		0.681
	Age	0.453	0.149	1.574	0.002 *
	Educational level	−0.043	0.157	0.958	0.78
	BMI	−0.160	0.155	0.852	0.302

* p value < 0.05 indicates significant comparison using chi-squared test.

3.5. Multiple Linear Regression Analysis

Multiple linear regression analysis was done to find the impact of three categorical independent variables, age, educational level and BMI, on four dependent outcomes, namely, general mental status, negative attitude, the impact of COVID-19 event and negative health impact. Table 5 shows age as a significant predictor for abnormal general mental status, development of negative attitude, eliciting impact of COVID-19 event and susceptibility to meet negative health impact. In addition to this, high bodyweight is another reason for altered mental status, negative attitude and developing impact of COVID-19 quickly. Overall, differences in the educational level have not shown any mental health impact.

4. Discussion

The difficult situation humanity is going through since the outbreak and declaration of the COVID-19 pandemic is unprecedented and unimaginable. The pandemic has adversely affected all walks of life, and every person on this earth has a direct or indirect impact. COVID-19 is a physical health problem, but it has the potential to cause a major mental health crisis if adequate and necessary steps are not taken in time. The World Health Organization recognized the implication of the COVID-19 pandemic on mental health and psychological functions and released a list of considerations to the public, health care workers, team leaders, and people under isolation and all other susceptible people to cut its impact [16]. Further, the United Nations proposed their recommendations to neutralize and combat the poor mental health outcomes by providing access to mental healthcare through creative means utilizing all other available and possible resources, especially across high-risk populations [17]. In addition to this, the Centers for Disease Control and Prevention (CDC) has shared measures and methods to overcome stress [18].

Although COVID-19 may produce altered mental health in any person, the section of the community vulnerable to mental alteration may get affected quickly. The mental health of all people of society is critical for the best functioning of the community. The well-being of the female population is a necessary element for the overall welfare of the system. Generally, women are more vulnerable to negative life events than men are, especially those without social support. A study carried out in Egypt reported a high prevalence of depression and anxiety in girls that are almost double that in boys [19]. In addition to this, there are several studies available in affirmation of the high incidence of mental abnormalities and quicker impact of events in females than men. Hence, the idea of this research to explain the impact of the ongoing pandemic on this vulnerable population of Riyadh, Saudi Arabia.

Overall, the mental status of the participant indicated mild alteration; however, around 44% of the participants acknowledge perceived depression due to the COVID-19 outbreak. The higher incidence of perceived depression in Saudi Arabian women is in accordance with the current global scenario [20]. People are continuously under fear of contracting infection, dying, and losing family members. Frequent misinformation through social media and other communication channels and nightmares about the future are common factors for the induction of depression. Possibly there is a role of organic changes in the central nervous system during the COVID-19 outbreak [21].

The psychological burden and alteration in mental status is a common feature of traumatic events. Studies done earlier have shown the negative implication of large scale traumatic events on the mental illness in the majority of vulnerable populations [22]. Additionally, the presence of co-morbid or riskier conditions may further enhance the impact of events. The impact of event scale-revised (IES-R) is one of the suitable scales subjectively measure the traumatic event such as COVID-19, especially in the response sets of intrusion (intrusive thoughts, nightmares, intrusive feelings and imagery, dissociative-like reexperiencing), avoidance (numbing of responsiveness, avoidance of feelings, situations, and ideas), and hyperarousal (anger, irritability, hypervigilance, difficulty concentrating, heightened startle), as well as total subjective stress IES-R score. The average score of this scale in our study showed a milder impact on the majority of the respondents, with an overall average of around 21. However, higher age groups and people of excess body weight have shown greater vulnerability to the COVID-19. The outcome of this study is in accordance with other studies reported earlier [10]. It is also interesting to note that the overall impact of the event was mild; however, 57% of the respondents still expressed added stress due to the pandemic, and 63% of them also feel apprehensive due to continuous reports of the pandemic. Probably, high stress and apprehension were due to the daily report of 2000–5000 new cases from the Kingdom of Saudi Arabia during the time of this study. Our findings are also consistent with other published literature showing that having exposure to life stressors are directly associated with more depression during times of social isolation as well as at low-intensity periods [23–25]. In addition to the adverse impact of COVID-19 on the economy of the country, an individual's economic status is also adversely affected due to the pandemic in many countries. However, the government of Saudi Arabia took exceptional care for the economic well-being of their citizens by facilitating full salaries and wages in both the public sector and the private sector. Hence, in our study, we did not notice any significant effect of COVID-19 associated economic status on the psychological burden of the participants.

To the best of our knowledge, our study was one of the few studies that have given insights about the extent of mental disturbance experienced by the feminine gender of the Saudi Arabia population living in the capital city, Riyadh, due to the COVID-19 pandemic. Additionally, it covered several parameters of measurement of mental status ranging from general health status to negative attitude, negative impact as well as the overall impact of COVID-19 using a reliable measuring tool.

However, it is an advantage to get to know the mental status of the female population. Having the data on the male gender would have help in comparing the extent of difference between the two sets of the population. Since most parts of this study were carried out during the lockdown phase, most of the respondents were reached through the social media link. There was no support offered to the participants on the tricky questions that need clarification that may count for understanding or interpretation bias on the part of the respondents. With a high percentage of the respondents having depression (44%), stress (53%) and apprehension (63%), it would be a good idea to do a large-scale study across different regions of the Kingdom of Saudi Arabia. Further, having data on the specific aspect of COVID-19, such as loss of a job, death of some beloved ones in the family, and others, could have given more insight into the specific issues. Additionally, as the number of cases dropping down in the Kingdom, the latest research will be needed to assess the trajectory of depression in the Saudi population and develop the potential treatment for affected populations.

5. Conclusions

The COVID-19 pandemic is associated with stress (53%), anxiety (63%) and depression (44%) in our sample population. Participants in the higher age group and overweight people have a high risk for alteration in mental health. Large scale study spread across different regions of Saudi Arabia, covering several types of population needed to assess the trajectory of the mental health of the Saudi population.

Author Contributions: Conceptualization, S.M.B.A.; data curation, S.A.A.; funding acquisition, Y.M.; methodology, M.A.; project administration, A.A.; resources, A.A.A.; supervision, S.M.B.A.; validation, S.N.; writing—original draft, N.N. All authors have read and agreed to the published version of the manuscript.

Funding: The authors would like to thank the Research Center at King Fahd Medical City, Riyadh, for their financial support provided for the manuscript.

Acknowledgments: The authors are thankful to AlMaarefa University, Riyadh, for providing support to do this research.

Conflicts of Interest: The authors declare no conflict of interest.

References

1. Kunin, M.; Engelhard, D.; Piterman, L.; Thomas, S. Response of general practitioners to infectious disease public health crises: An integrative systematic review of the literature. *Disaster Med. Public Health Prep.* **2013**, *7*, 522–533. [CrossRef] [PubMed]
2. Panchal, N.; Kamal, R.; Orgera, K.; Cox, C.; Garfield, R.; Hamel, L.; Chidambaram, P. The Implications of COVID-19 for Mental Health and Substance use. Available online: https://www.kff.org/coronavirus-covid-19/issue-brief/the-implications-of-covid-19-for-mental-health-and-substance-use/ (accessed on 5 April 2020).
3. WHO. Mental Health & COVID-19. Available online: https://www.who.int/teams/mental-health-and-substance-use/covid-19 (accessed on 19 September 2020).
4. Pfefferbaum, B.; North, C.S. Mental health and the Covid-19 pandemic. *N. Engl. J. Med.* **2020**, *383*, 510–512. [CrossRef]
5. Szmuda, T.; Ali, S.; Słoniewski, P. Telemedicine in neurosurgery during the novel coronavirus (COVID-19) pandemic. *Neurol. Neurochir. Pol.* **2020**, *54*, 207–208. [PubMed]
6. Asdaq, S.M.; Yasmin, F. Risk of psychological burden in polycystic ovary syndrome: A case control study in Riyadh, Saudi Arabia. *J. Affect. Disord.* **2020**, *274*, 205–209. [CrossRef]
7. PAHO/WHO. *Protecting Mental Health during Epidemics*; PAHO/WHO: Washington, DC, USA, 2005.
8. Nguyen, L.H.; Drew, D.A.; Graham, M.S.; Joshi, A.D.; Guo, C.G.; Ma, W.; Mehta, R.S.; Warner, E.T.; Sikavi, D.R.; Lo, C.H.; et al. Risk of COVID-19 among front-line health-care workers and the general community: A prospective cohort study. *Lancet Public Health* **2020**, *5*, e475–e483. [CrossRef]
9. Ahmed, H.; Allaf, M.; Elghazaly, H. COVID-19 and medical education. *Lancet Infect. Dis.* **2020**, *20*, 777–778. [CrossRef]
10. Zhang, Y.; Ma, Z.F. Impact of the COVID-19 pandemic on mental health and quality of life among local residents in Liaoning Province, China: A cross-sectional study. *Int. J. Environ. Res. Public Health* **2020**, *17*, 2381. [CrossRef]
11. Alghadeer, S.M.; Alhossan, A.M.; Al-Arifi, M.N.; Alrabiah, Z.S.; Ali, S.W.; Babelghaith, S.D.; Altamimi, M.A. Prevalence of mental disorders among patients attending primary health care centers in the capital of Saudi Arabia. *Neurosciences* **2018**, *23*, 238–243. [CrossRef] [PubMed]
12. Zatzick, D.F.; Marmar, C.R.; Weiss, D.S.; Browner, W.S.; Metzler, T.J.; Golding, J.M.; Stewart, A.; Schlenger, W.E.; Wells, K.B. Posttraumatic stress disorder and functioning and quality of life outcomes in a nationally representative sample of male Vietnam veterans. *Am. J. Psychiatry* **1997**, *154*, 1690–1695. [CrossRef] [PubMed]
13. Beck, J.; Grant, D.; Read, J.; Clapp, J.; Coffey, S.; Miller, L.; Palyo, S. The Impact of Event Scale-Revised: Psychometric properties in a sample of motor vehicle accident survivors. *J. Anxiety Disord.* **2008**, *22*, 187–198. [CrossRef] [PubMed]
14. Dyregrov, A.; Gjestad, R. A maritime disaster: Reactions and follow-up. *Int. J. Emerg. Ment. Health* **2003**, *5*, 3–14. [PubMed]
15. Lau, J.T.; Yang, X.; Tsui, H.Y.; Pang, E.; Wing, Y.K. Positive mental health-related impacts of the sars epidemic on the general public in hong kong and their associations with other negative impacts. *J. Infect.* **2006**, *53*, 114–124. [CrossRef] [PubMed]
16. World Health Organization. Mental Health and Psychosocial Considerations during the COVID-19 Outbreak. WHO/2019-nCoV/MentalHealth/2020.1. 2020. Available online: https://www.who.int/docs/default-source/coronaviruse/mental-health-considerations.pdf (accessed on 10 April 2020).
17. United Nations Policy Brief: Covid-19 and the Need for Action on Mental Health. Available online: https://www.un.org/sites/un2.un.org/files/un_policy_brief-covid_and_mental_health_final.pdf (accessed on 10 April 2020).
18. Centers for Disease Control and Prevention. Available online: https://www.cdc.gov/coronavirus/2019-ncov/daily-life-coping/managing-stress-anxiety.html?CDC_AA_refVal=https%3A%2F%2Fwww.cdc.gov%2Fcoronavirus%2F2019-ncov%2Fprepare%2Fmanaging-stress-anxiety.html (accessed on 15 April 2020).
19. Afifi, M. Depression in adolescents: Gender differences in Oman and Egypt. *East. Mediterr. Health J.* **2006**, *12*, 61–71. [PubMed]
20. Ettman, C.K.; Abdalla, S.M.; Cohen, G.H.; Sampson, L.; Vivier, P.M.; Galea, S. Prevalence of Depression Symptoms in US Adults Before and During the COVID-19 Pandemic. *JAMA Netw. Open* **2020**, *3*, e2019686. [CrossRef] [PubMed]

21. Słyk, S.; Domitrz, I. Neurological manifestations of SARS-CoV-2—A systematic review. *Neurol. Neurochir. Pol.* **2020**, *54*, 378–383. [CrossRef] [PubMed]
22. Goldmann, E.; Galea, S. Mental health consequences of disasters. *Annu. Rev. Public Health* **2014**, *35*, 169–183. [CrossRef] [PubMed]
23. Cronkite, R.C.; Woodhead, E.L.; Finlay, A.; Timko, C.; Unger Hu, K.; Moos, R.H. Life stressors and resources and the 23-year course of depression. *J. Affect. Disord.* **2013**, *150*, 370–377. [CrossRef] [PubMed]
24. Kessler, R.C. The effects of stressful life events on depression. *Annu. Rev. Psychol.* **1997**, *48*, 191–214. [CrossRef] [PubMed]
25. McAllister, A.; Fritzell, S.; Almroth, M.; Harber-Aschan, L.; Larsson, S.; Burström, B. How do macro-level structural determinants affect inequalities in mental health: A systematic review of the literature. *Int. J. Equity Health* **2018**, *17*, 180. [CrossRef] [PubMed]

Publisher's Note: MDPI stays neutral with regard to jurisdictional claims in published maps and institutional affiliations.

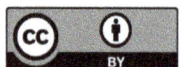

© 2020 by the authors. Licensee MDPI, Basel, Switzerland. This article is an open access article distributed under the terms and conditions of the Creative Commons Attribution (CC BY) license (http://creativecommons.org/licenses/by/4.0/).

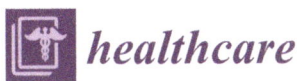

Article

Associations between Personality Traits, Intolerance of Uncertainty, Coping Strategies, and Stress in Italian Frontline and Non-Frontline HCWs during the COVID-19 Pandemic—A Multi-Group Path-Analysis

Ramona Bongelli [1,*], Carla Canestrari [2], Alessandra Fermani [2], Morena Muzi [2], Ilaria Riccioni [2], Alessia Bertolazzi [1] and Roberto Burro [3]

1. Department of Political Science, Communication and International Relations, University of Macerata, 62100 Macerata, Italy; alessia.bertolazzi@unimc.it
2. Department of Education, Cultural Heritage and Tourism, University of Macerata, 62100 Macerata, Italy; carla.canestrari@unimc.it (C.C.); alessandra.fermani@unimc.it (A.F.); morena.muzi@unimc.it (M.M.); ilaria.riccioni@unimc.it (I.R.)
3. Department of Human Sciences, University of Verona, 37129 Verona, Italy; roberto.burro@univr.it
* Correspondence: ramona.bongelli@unimc.it; Tel.: +39-0733-2582540

Citation: Bongelli, R.; Canestrari, C.; Fermani, A.; Muzi, M.; Riccioni, I.; Bertolazzi, A.; Burro, R. Associations between Personality Traits, Intolerance of Uncertainty, Coping Strategies, and Stress in Italian Frontline and Non-Frontline HCWs during the COVID-19 Pandemic—A Multi-Group Path-Analysis. *Healthcare* **2021**, *9*, 1086. https://doi.org/10.3390/healthcare9081086

Academic Editors: Manoj Sharma and Kavita Batra

Received: 30 July 2021
Accepted: 18 August 2021
Published: 23 August 2021

Publisher's Note: MDPI stays neutral with regard to jurisdictional claims in published maps and institutional affiliations.

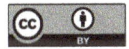

Copyright: © 2021 by the authors. Licensee MDPI, Basel, Switzerland. This article is an open access article distributed under the terms and conditions of the Creative Commons Attribution (CC BY) license (https://creativecommons.org/licenses/by/4.0/).

Abstract: The COVID-19 pandemic represented a very difficult physical and psychological challenge for the general population and even more for healthcare workers (HCWs). The main aim of the present study is to test whether there were significant differences between frontline and non-frontline Italian HCWs concerning (a) personality traits, intolerance of uncertainty, coping strategies and perceived stress, and (b) the models of their associations. A total of 682 Italian HCWs completed a self-report questionnaire: 280 employed in COVID-19 wards and 402 in other wards. The analysis of variance omnibus test revealed significant differences between the two groups only for perceived stress, which was higher among the frontline. The multi-group path analysis revealed significant differences in the structure of the associations between the two groups of HCWs, specifically concerning the relations between: personality traits and intolerance of uncertainty; intolerance of uncertainty and coping strategies. Regarding the relation between coping strategies and stress no difference was identified between the two groups. In both of them, emotionally focused coping was negatively related with perceived stress, whereas dysfunctional coping was positively related with stress. These results could be useful in planning actions aiming to reduce stress and improve the effectiveness of HCWs' interventions. Training programs aimed to provide HCWs with a skillset to tackle uncertain and stressful circumstances could represent an appropriate support to develop a preventive approach during outbreaks.

Keywords: COVID-19; HCWs; personality traits; intolerance of uncertainty; coping strategies; perceived stress

1. Introduction

The COVID-19 pandemic is undoubtedly one of the greatest disasters of the 21st century for people all over the world. The pandemic is a very serious threat, both physical and psychological, for the general population [1–5], but even more for vulnerable groups of subjects. The latter include, among others, patients with pre-existent mental health disorders, as well as those suffering from other chronic or acute diseases, such as cancer patients. While COVID-19 and the related strict lockdown caused, since the first wave of the pandemic, severe psychological effects (such as relapses, worsening of conditions, stress, anger, impulsivity, etc., e.g., [6–9]) on patients suffering from mental disorders, it has been particularly challenging also for cancer patients, who are at a high risk of contracting the virus and of developing more severe complications compared to the general population [10].

Thus, the fear of being infected makes the COVID-19 a new stressor [11], able to affect their emotional and social functioning [12].

At the same time, the COVID-19 pandemic represents a very arduous challenge for both the scientific community—involved in finding vaccines to prevent its spread, and therapies to cure infected people [13]—and healthcare workers (HCWs) —who, working daily in facing it, not only jeopardize their own physical health (risking to get infected), but also their mental wellbeing. Consistently with the results of many studies on the psychological impact of past pandemics on health professionals [14–16], the literature published until now about COVID-19 revealed that HCWs are at particular risk of adverse psychological outcomes, i.e., of developing more severe mental symptoms, including stress, anxiety, depression, distress, insomnia, emotional exhaustion, burnout, as well as post-traumatic stress disorder [17–40]. These adverse consequences regard specifically those working on the frontline [17] (i.e., those directly engaged in the diagnosis, treatment, and care for patients with COVID-19, employed in emergency departments, intensive care units, and infectious disease wards) and in areas (such as China and Italy) where the virus has had a rapid spread and caused a high number of hospitalizations (in intensive care units) and deaths (especially during the first months of its circulation).

These negative psychological outcomes on HCWSs are undoubtedly related to the situation—that, specifically during the first wave of the virus spread, was in itself particularly demanding [24], stressful, and characterized by high levels of uncertainty—but probably also to more specific contextual conditions (first of all, as argued above, having worked on the frontline or not), as well as to individual differences, such as HCWs' personality traits (that are "one of the important determinants for the development of mental health issues during the pandemic situation" [41] (p. 5)), ability to tolerate uncertainty, and to cope with the situation.

1.1. Intolerance of Uncertainty, Personality, and Coping

All pandemics, including the one caused by COVID-19, being unexpected and unpredictable events, which affect large numbers of people, are sources of stress (i.e., they are cataclysmic stressors, according to Lazarus and Cohen's definition [42]), and uncertainty among both ordinary people and HCWs [43–45]. If ordinary people experience "uncertainty about getting infected, uncertainty about the seriousness of the infection, uncertainty about whether the people around you are infected, uncertainty about whether objects or surfaces (e.g., money, doorknobs) are infected, uncertainty about the optimal type of treatment or protective measures, and uncertainty about whether a pandemic is truly over" [44] (p. 43), HCWs experience also other types of uncertainty (both professional and personal), that differ during the different stages of virus diffusion. Among them, uncertainty about how dangerous and contagious the virus is, uncertainty about therapies and cures, uncertainty concerning personal devices to be adopted in order to avoid getting infected while working (and become a vehicle of infection for other people, e.g. patients or relatives), uncertainties about the right measures for containing the virus spread (e.g., use of masks and gloves), etc.

Although uncertainty during a pandemic is, therefore, a common experience for everybody, including HCWs, nonetheless the individuals' abilities to tolerate it varies greatly. Some people, more than others, show indeed more difficulty in tolerating uncertainty.

Intolerance of uncertainty can be defined as a dispositional fear of the unknown [46–48], which seems to be related to certain personality traits [49], specifically to neuroticism (or negative emotionality, which is one of the five personality traits identified by the BIG Five Model [50]; see Section 2.2. "Measures"). It can be considered as a sub-trait of anxiety [44] (that is, in its turn, a facet of neuroticism), which has often been found in association with stress, distress, insomnia, psychosomatic symptoms, and other clinical conditions in several recent studies carried out on COVID-19 among the general population and HCWs (e.g., [45,51–56]). It is a cognitive, emotional, and behavioral tendency to react negatively to uncertain or ambiguous situations and unpredictable future events [57,58], which biases information processing, leading to faulty appraisals of threat, and reduces coping abilities [59].

1.2. Coping, Personality, Intolerance of Uncertainty

Coping, in its turn, can be defined as the set of cognitive and behavioral efforts to manage specific external and/or internal demands, which are evaluated as taxing or exceeding a person's resources [60] or, more simply, as processes of response to stressors [61]. Like Monzani et al. [62] state, coping strategies have been classified differently, mainly in dichotomous pairs, by different authors: problem-focused, (i.e., aiming at actively responding to a stressful situation) vs. emotion-focused coping (i.e., aiming to reduce or manage emotions related to the stressful situation) [63,64]; approach, (i.e., aiming to directly face with stressors and related emotions) vs. avoidance strategies (i.e., aiming to deny, minimize, or avoid dealing with stressors) [65–67]; adaptive (i.e., characterized by more probability of obtaining a result) vs. ineffective or maladaptive (i.e., characterized by more probability of not obtaining a result) [67,68]).

The vast literature on this topic revealed that the use of coping strategies is influenced by many variables, among which are situational demands, environmental and cultural aspects, personal characters [63], as well as individuals' ability to tolerate uncertainty [59], and personality traits [69–71]. In other terms, different persons, in different situations, resort to different coping strategies.

Many recent studies during the COVID-19 pandemic have been conducted in different contexts among both the general population and health professionals, showing great variability in the use of coping strategies. Taylor et al. [72], for example, revealed that during the lockdown, people have found many different ways of making self-isolation more tolerable, which include watching TV or movies. Regarding HCWs, Munawar and Choundry [73], for example, identified different types of coping strategies used by Malaysian HCWs to deal with stress and anxiety, but one of the most recurring was the religion coping strategy. Salman et al. [74] found, in a sample of HCWs from Pakistan, that positive coping strategies were more widely used than avoidant and maladaptive strategies. Huang et al. [75], comparing nurses with nursing students, found that the former use more problem-focused coping strategies than the latter.

As mentioned above, the use of different coping strategies is not only linked to specific contextual, environmental, or cultural conditions, it also seems to be influenced by individuals' dispositional traits. As for the link between coping strategies and intolerance of uncertainty, although much research has been conducted revealing clear associations between them [59], as far as we know, few studies focused on the relations between intolerance of uncertainty and coping strategies during a pandemic and none of them explicitly analyzed this relation in samples of HCWs. One of the best-known research about intolerance of uncertainty and coping was the one conducted by Taha et al. [76] in a general population sample during the H1N1 pandemic of 2009. The authors found significant relations between, greater intolerance of uncertainty, on the one hand, and lower problem-focused and higher emotion-focused coping strategies, on the other. Instead, Rettie and Daniels [77], studying a sample of the general population during the COVID-19 pandemic, found that maladaptive coping strategies mediate the relationship between intolerance of uncertainty and distress.

As far as coping strategies and personality are concerned (see Section 2.2 for the personality traits), scientific research not only revealed that personality influences the way people cope with stressful situations, but identified also specific relations between them. For example, according to Leandro and Castillo [70], and Afshar et al. [71], maladaptive personality traits (e.g., neuroticism) positively correlate with emotion-focused and avoidant (dysfunctional) coping strategies; on the contrary, extraversion positively correlates with problem-focused and emotional-focused strategies [69]. Several recent studies on COVID-19 have also identified similar links between personality traits and adaptive and maladaptive coping responses. Sica et al. [78], for example, found, in a sample of

Italian adults, positive association between maladaptive traits of personality and avoidant forms of coping (e.g., drug use), and negative associations between maladaptive traits and acceptance and positive reframing. Other studies have not only substantially confirmed these results, but have also found significant associations with the levels of perceived stress. According to Liu et al. [79], for example, individuals with higher levels of neuroticism would have the tendency "to perceive events as highly threatening and often have limited coping resources, self-regulation and perceived efficacy, and thus resulting in a higher level of stress" [79] (p. 2). Conversely, people with high levels of conscientiousness seem to be able to resort to more effective coping strategies, thus experiencing lower levels of stress.

1.3. Current Study

Consistently with the results of the literature on the topic, it seems reasonable to assume that specific contextual situations as well as some individual characteristics—i.e., personality traits, intolerance of uncertainty, coping strategies—have specific relations among them and differently impact on psychological outcomes, specifically on perceived stress. Nonetheless, to the best of our knowledge, no study has been conducted to explicitly investigate these associations in samples of HCWs during the COVID-19 pandemic.

Thus, also considering the great amount of work, under uncertain and stressful conditions, the present study aimed at investigating, in a sample of Italian HCWs, employed during the first wave of the COVID-19 pandemic, the relations between some personal characteristics and perceived stress, by testing whether the variable "having worked on the frontline" (i.e., in a COVID dedicated ward) or "not having worked on the frontline" (i.e., in other wards) affects them (i.e., affects the relations between the variables taken into account).

The analyses revealed significant differences both in the levels of perceived stress, which were higher in the frontline HCWs than in the non-frontline, and in the structure of the associations between the two groups, specifically concerning the relations between: personality traits and intolerance of uncertainty; intolerance of uncertainty and coping strategies. Regarding the relations between coping strategies and stress, no difference was identified. In both groups, the use of emotional coping strategies was linked indeed to lower levels of perceived stress, while the use of dysfunctional coping strategies to higher levels of perceived stress.

2. Methods

2.1. Data Collection

This study, conducted according to Helsinki Declaration principles (https://www.wma.net/what-we-do/medical-ethics/declaration-of-helsinki/, accessed on 22 August 2021), APA Ethics Code, and European and Italian Privacy Law (i.e., EU Reg. 679/2016, GDPRD and Legislative Decree n. 196/2003, Code regarding the protection of personal data), has been approved by PhD meeting curriculum in Psychology, Communication, and Social Sciences, (University of Macerata. Protocol code n. 19435, 3 August 2020).

It was conducted through an online survey, which started on May 15 and ended on 30 July 2020, to which Italian HCWs (nurses and physicians), enrolled in professional orders and associations, were invited to participate. The snowball sampling method was used.

Specifically, during the first week of May 2020, the authors sent an email to the presidents of all the Italian orders of physicians and nurses and of the main professional associations (e.g., Associazione Anestesisti Rianimatori Ospedalieri Italiani emergenza area critica/Italian Hospital Anesthetist Association for critical area emergency) to present the research protocol and asked them to send an invitation email to their members with the link to compile a self-report questionnaire or to publish it on their website. After three weeks, the authors sent a reminder email to those orders and associations that did not respond to the first email.

It should be noted that before sending the emails and making public the link to the online survey, three physicians, one obstetrician, and one nurse compiled the questionnaire and provided the authors their favorable opinion regarding its length, clarity, and comprehensibility of all the items. Survey administration was conducted through LimeSurvey software on a LAMP (Linux, Apache, MySQL, PHP, a common example of a web service stack) server. All communication was encrypted, using HTTPS protocol and Secure Sockets Layer (SSL). No prize, as an incentive to compile the survey was offered, since it is not common practice in Italy and it could also affect the data by inducing subjects to offer socially desirable answers, thus compromising data reliability.

The questionnaire opened with some information concerning the aims of the research, the identity and contacts of the research team, the planned ways of disseminating the results, the references to the European and Italian privacy laws, and protection of personal data. The respondents could begin to fill in the questionnaire after having voluntarily consented to participate by signing an online informed consent. The questionnaire was composed of:

- Twelve questions, aiming to collect socio-demographic, employment information, and information concerning the exposure of HCWs to COVID-19;
- Four validated scales (see Section 2.2. "Measures"), aiming to measure HCWs' personality traits, intolerance of uncertainty, coping strategies, and perceived stress;
- One final open-ended question (which is not taken into account in the present study, as it is the specific subject of another paper that we are going to submit), aiming to know whether and how the experience of having worked during the pandemic had an emotional impact on HCWs.

All the items of the questionnaire were compulsory, except for the open-ended question. The estimated average time for compiling the questionnaire was approximately 15 min.

2.2. Measures

2.2.1. Personal Information Data

In order to collect socio-demographic and job characteristics, as well as more specific information concerning their exposure to COVID-19, HCWs were asked questions concerning gender, age, marital and parental status, religion, job position (doctor or nurse), specialties (area), place of work, seniority, job exposure to COVID-19, COVID-19 swabs (i.e., having received swabs for COVID-19), and contraction of COVID-19.

2.2.2. Big Five Inventory, Short Version (BFI-2-S)

The Italian HCWs' personality trait domains were assessed using the Italian translation of the 30-item BFI-2-S [80]; it is a short version of the 60-item BFI-2 [81], which, in its turn, represents a revision of the Big Five Inventory (BFI, [82–84]).

The BFI-2 "operationalizes the hierarchical conceptualization of personality structure by assessing the Big Five domains and 15 facets: Extraversion (with facets of Sociability, Assertiveness, and Energy Level), Agreeableness (Compassion, Respectfulness, and Trust), Conscientiousness (Organization, Productiveness, and Responsibility), Negative Emotionality (Anxiety, Depression, and Emotional Volatility), and Open-Mindedness (Intellectual Curiosity, Aesthetic Sensitivity, and Creative Imagination)" [81] (p. 69). Respondents rate each of the 30 items using a five-point scale ranging from 1 (strongly disagree) to 5 (strongly agree).

The CFA outcomes supported the hypothesized structure: all standardized factor loadings resulted statistically significant (with values between 0.420 and 0.914), and the goodness of fit indexes acceptable (CFI = 0.911; TLI = 0.902; RMSEA = 0.079; SRMR = 0.088). We considered (throughout the article) as fit indexes the comparative fit index (CFI), the TLI, the RMSEA, and the SRMR, with CFI and TLI ≥ 0.90, RMSEA ≤ 0.08, and SRMR ≤ 0.06 as threshold values [85].

Cronbach's alpha and McDonald's omega were respectively 0.74 and 0.73 for Extraversion, 0.71 and 0.70 for Agreeableness, 0.70 and 0.69 for Conscientiousness, 0.77 and 0.77 for Negative Emotionality, 0.77 and 0.78 for Open-Mindedness.

2.2.3. Intolerance of Uncertainty Scale (IUS-12)

The Italian HCWs' intolerance of uncertainty was assessed using the Italian version [86] of IUS-12 [87]; it is the short version of the 27-item intolerance of uncertainty scale (IUS-27 [88]), developed to evaluate "emotional, cognitive and behavioral reactions to ambiguous situations, implications of being uncertain, and attempts to control the future" [88] (p. 791). IUS-12 is a two-factor scale that represents two different sub-dimensions of intolerance toward uncertainty: prospective and inhibitory [49,87]. The former reflects "desire for predictability and active engagement in information seeking to increase certainty"; the latter reflects "uncertainty avoidance and paralysis in the face of uncertainty" [89] (p. 377). Respondents assess the items on a five-point Likert scale, ranging from 1 (not at all characteristic of me) to 5 (entirely characteristic of me).

Both the Cronbach's alpha and McDonald's omega were 0.90 for the overall scale; Cronbach's alpha for prospective intolerance of uncertainty (items 1–7) was 0.83 and McDonald's omega was 0.84, while alpha and omega for inhibitory intolerance (items 8–12) were 0.90.

2.2.4. Brief-COPE Scale

The Italian HCWs' coping strategies were evaluated using the Brief-COPE [66]; it is the short version of the original COPE (Coping Orientation to Problems Experienced) inventory [65]. We adapted the original Brief-COPE scale into the Italian language using a forward and backward translation process to guarantee correspondence between Italian and English original versions. The Brief-COPE consists of 14 faced-scales (each of them composed of 2 items), which represent 14 different coping strategies [66,67] that can be grouped into two overarching coping styles: approach coping (active coping, planning, positive reframing, acceptance, seeking emotional support, seeking instrumental support) and avoidant coping (self-distraction, denial, venting, substance use, behavioral disengagement, self-blame). Humor and religion are excluded from these styles, since, according to [90], they are both adaptive and problematic components. Some authors (e.g., [63]) distinguish the 14 faced-scales into three composite subscales: problem-focused (active coping, seeking instrumental support, planning), emotion-focused (acceptance, seeking emotional support, humor, positive reframing, religion), and dysfunctional (behavioral disengagement, denial, self-blame, self-distraction, substance use, venting). The 28 items, that are measured with scores ranging from 0 (I haven't been doing this at all) to 3 (I've been doing this a lot), can be "converted to a dispositional 'coping style' format [...] or a situational concurrent format, by changing verb forms [...]. They can assume a retrospective, situational format [...], a concurrent situational format [...], or even a dispositional format" [66] (pp. 95–98). Since we wanted to measure the Italian healthcare professionals' situational and retrospective coping strategies, i.e., related to a specific circumstance (the COVID-19 pandemic), we presented the items in the past tense.

In order to assess the goodness of fit indexes of the factor structure of the Italian version of the Brief-COPE scale, we performed a Confirmatory Factor Analysis (CFA). The CFA outcomes supported the hypothesized structure: all standardized factor loadings resulted statistically significant (with values between 0.430 and 0.989), and the goodness of fit indexes acceptable (CFI = 0.927; TLI = 0.919; RMSEA = 0.078; SRMR = 0.089).

Cronbach alpha for the Brief-COPE was 0.82, and McDonald's omega was 0.82. Specifically, following the distinction between problem-focused, emotion-focused, and dysfunctional strategies, we obtained that alpha and omega for problem-focused strategies were 0.76 and 0.77, respectively, while for emotion-focused strategies 0.71 and 0.77, respectively. Alpha and omega for dysfunctional strategies were 0.77 and 0.79, respectively.

2.2.5. Italian Perceived Stress Scale (IPSS-10)

The Italian HCWs' perceived stress was measured using the IPSS-10 (Italian Perceived Stress Scale); it is the Italian version [91] of the PSS (Perceived stress scale). Although its original version consists of 14 items [92], the most commonly used is that consisting of

10 items [93,94]. PSS measures the degree to which situations in one's life are evaluated as stressful [95] (p. 1) by asking about feelings and thoughts during the last month. Respondents are asked how often they felt a certain way on a five-point Likert scale: 0 = Never; 1 = Almost Never; 2 = Sometimes; 3 = Fairly Often; 4 = Very Often. Cronbach's alpha was 0.881 and McDonald's omega 0.884.

2.3. Procedures

In order to investigate the associations between personality traits, intolerance of uncertainty, coping strategies and perceived stress in a sample of Italian HCWs, also taking into account different situational contexts (i.e., having worked on the frontline or not), we

a. First, tested if there were significant differences between the two groups of HCWs (frontline and non-frontline) in relation to each of the variables considered;
b. Second, developed and tested a model (see Figure 1), according to which personality traits can differentially impact on intolerance of uncertainty, intolerance of uncertainty can differently impact on the use of coping strategies, and coping strategies can differently affect the level of perceived stress;
c. Finally, tested whether the structure of the relations (see Figure 1) vary in the two groups of HCWs.

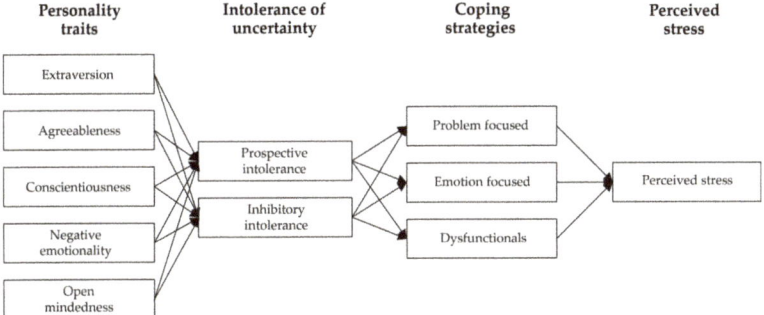

Figure 1. Path-diagram of the general model of structure of relations among variables.

2.4. Data Analysis

Descriptive statistics (n, %) were conducted, using the R-software (version 4.1.0, [96]), to have a complete picture of our sample.

In order to determine whether there were significant differences between frontline and non-frontline HCWs, three different linear mixed models (LMMs) were applied using personality traits (based on BFI-2-S score), intolerance of uncertainty (based on IUS-12 score), and coping strategies (emotional focused, problem focused, avoidant; based on Brief-COPE score) as fixed effects, and subject ID as random effect. A linear model (LM) was performed for perceived stress (based on IPSS-10). Three analyses of variance fixed effects omnibus tests (regarding LMMs), and one analysis of variance omnibus test (regarding LM) were calculated.

A multi-group path-analysis was performed, using lavaan R software package [97], in order to test whether having worked in a dedicated COVID ward or not during the first wave of the pandemic in Italy would have determined differences in the associations (i.e., in the structure of relations) between personality traits, intolerance of uncertainty, coping strategies, and perceived stress.

3. Results

3.1. Sample Characteristics

Out of 682 participants who fully compiled the questionnaire, 530 (77.71%) were women and 152 (22.29%) men. The participants' answers contained no missing data (answers to individual questions were mandatory to complete the questionnaire). Incomplete questionnaires were not taken into account. The mean age was 45.39 (ranging from 21 to 81, SD = 12.04). The majority of them were married (44.36%), had children (57.92%), declared to be religious persons (practitioners: 15.84%; non-practitioners: 23.75%; only occasional practitioners: 38.42%). Furthermore, 75.95% worked as a nurse, 70.23% in hospitals and care services in the northern region of Italy, 51.76% in the area of medical specialties, with 47.65% working for more than 20 years. Moreover, 41.06% of them claimed to have worked in a COVID-19-dedicated ward, i.e., on the frontline, while 58.94% in other wards. Although more than half of them (57.48%) had a swab test for COVID-19, fortunately, only a low percentage contracted the virus (8.36%). The following Table 1 shows a more detailed description of our sample characteristics.

3.2. Analysis of Variance

The analysis of variance fixed effects omnibus test (Type III analysis of variance with Satterthwaite's method), conducted on the LMMs, revealed no significant differences between frontline and non-frontline HCWs concerning personality traits, $F(4, 2720) = 1.664$, $p = 0.155$ (see Figure 2A), intolerance of uncertainty, $F(1, 680) = 0.131$, $p = 0.718$ (see Figure 2B) and coping strategies, $F(1, 1360) = 2.253$, $p = 0.106$ (see Figure 3A).

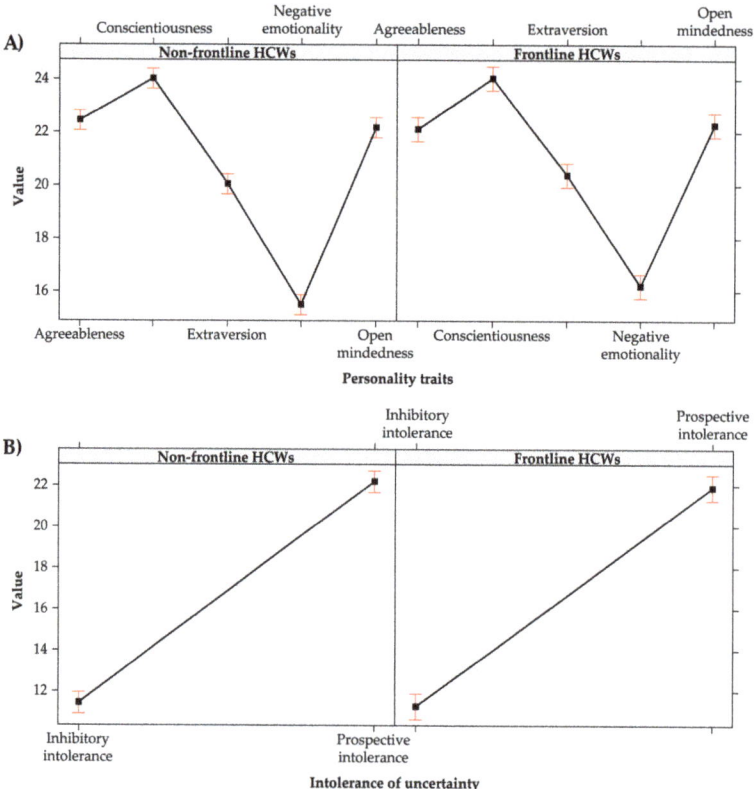

Figure 2. Effect plot of: (**A**) personality traits; (**B**) intolerance of uncertainly. The bars represent the 95% CI.

Table 1. Descriptive statistics of the sample characteristics.

Variables	n (%)
Total	682 (100.00%)
Socio-demographic characteristics	
Gender	
Female	530 (77.71%)
Male	152 (22.29%)
Age	
18–30	128 (18.77%)
31–40	131 (19.21%)
41–50	182 (26.69%)
51–60	193 (28.30%)
>60	48 (7.04%)
Marital status	
Married	307 (45.01%)
Unmarried	188 (27.57%)
Domestic partner	107 (15.69%)
Divorced/separated	67 (9.82%)
Widower/widow	13 (1.91%)
Children	
Yes	395 (57.92%)
No	287 (42.08%)
Religion	
Believer occasionally practitioner	262 (38.42%)
Believer non-practitioner	162 (23.75%)
Non-Believer	113 (16.57%)
Believer practitioner	108 (15.84%)
Prefer not to answer	37 (5.43%)
Job characteristics	
Place of work	
North Italy	479 (70.23%)
Centre Italy	128 (18.77%)
South Italy	75 (11.00%)
Job position	
Nurse	518 (75.95%)
Physician	164 (24.05%)
Job area	
Medical specialties	353 (51.76%)
Diagnostic and therapeutic specialties	144 (21.11%)
Surgical specialties	106 (15.54%)
Primary care nurse. serv.	79 (11.58%)
Seniority	
More than 20 years	325 (47.65%)
Less than 5 years	150 (21.99%)
10–20 years	121 (17.74%)
5–10 years	86 (12.61%)
Job exposure to COVID-19	
Wards	
Worked in COVID-19-dedicated wards	280 (41.06%)
Worked in other wards	402 (58.94%)
Swabs for COVID-19	
Done	392 (57.48%)
Not done	290 (42.52%)
COVID-19 contracted	
No	534 (78.30%)
Perhaps	91 (13.34%)
Yes	57 (8.36%)

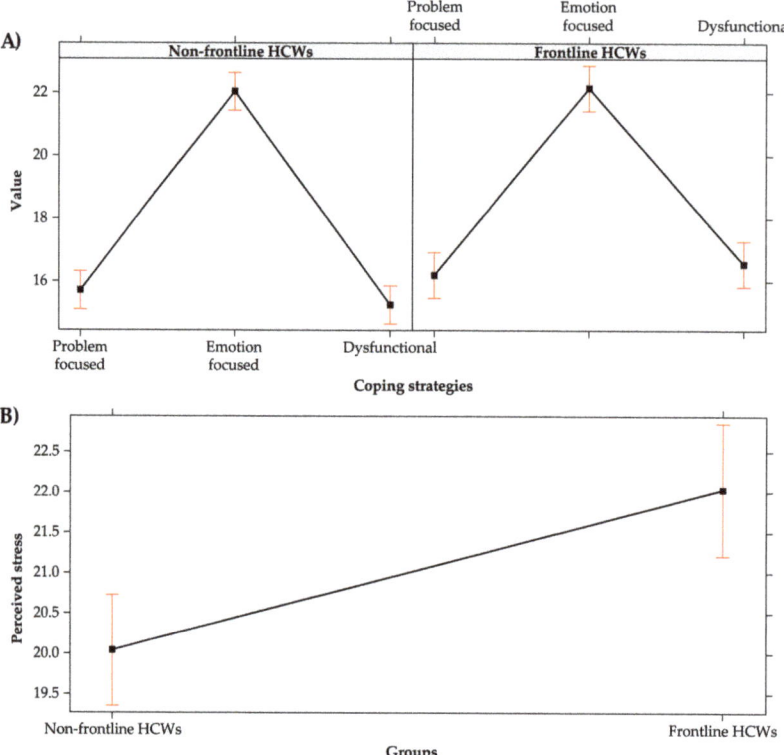

Figure 3. Effect plot of: (**A**) coping strategies; (**B**) perceived stress of groups. The bars represent the 95% CI.

In particular, in both groups of HCWs

- The conscientiousness (i.e., organization, productiveness, and responsibility) was the most prevalent personality trait;
- Levels of prospective intolerance of uncertainty were higher than the levels of inhibitory one;
- Emotion-focused coping strategies were more used than problem-focused and dysfunctional coping strategies.

On the contrary, the results of the analysis of variance omnibus test (Type III analysis of variance) conducted on the linear model (LM) revealed significant differences between the two groups about the perceived stress, $F(1, 680) = 9.394$, $p = 0.002$, Cohen's d = 0.240, i.e., the quantitative size of the estimated effect is closer to the small than to the medium value. Specifically, the levels of perceived stress were higher among the frontline Italian HCWs (M = 22.032, SD = 8.649, 95% CI [21.447, 22.617]) rather than among the non-frontline (M = 20.042, SD = 8.119, 95% CI [19.584, 20.501]) (see Figure 3B).

In Figure 4, we report the correlations and the descriptive statistics for personality traits, intolerance of uncertainly, coping strategies, and perceived stress.

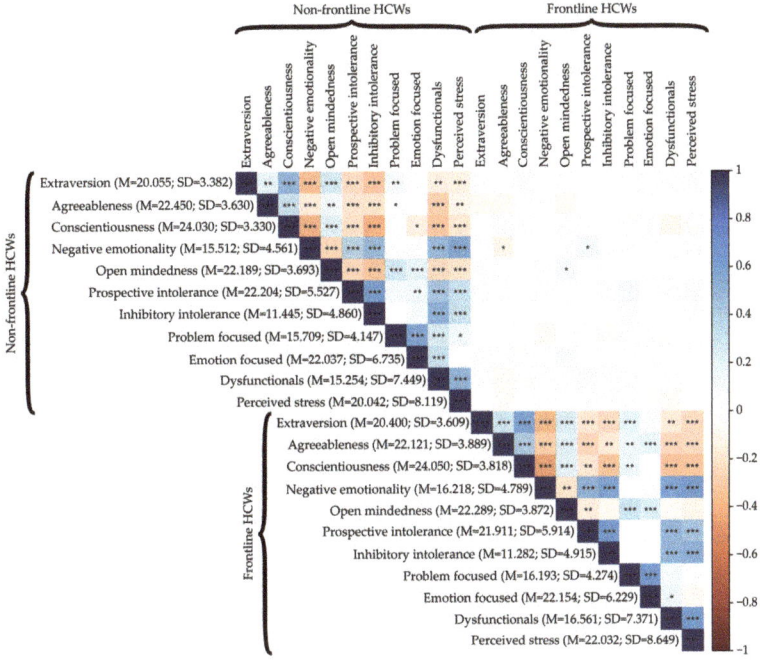

Figure 4. Pearson's Correlations and descriptive statistics of the experimental variables (* $p < 0.05$, ** $p < 0.01$, *** $p < 0.001$).

3.3. Multi-Group Path-Analysis

We ran the multi-group path-analysis (see path-diagram in Figure 1) using the "Diagonally Weighted Least Squares" (DWLS) estimator. For a proper analysis, the minimum ratio between the number of observations and the number of model parameters should be greater than 5:1 [85]. In our case, we had 110 estimated parameters with 682 participants, therefore the ratio was 6.2:1, and the sample size was adequate. We obtained adequate fit indices: CFI = 0.959, TLI = 0.917, RMSEA = 0.077, and SRMR = 0.060.

Using RMSEA as effect size and alpha = 0.05, the results of the post-hoc power analysis show that a sample size of N = 682 is associated with a power larger than 99.99%.

The Chi-squared difference test between the multi-group unconstrained and constrained models revealed significant differences (see Table 2) between Italian frontline and non-frontline HCWs concerning the associations (structure of the relations) among personality traits, intolerance of uncertainty, coping strategies, and perceived stress.

Table 2. Differences between frontline and non-frontline HCWs.

Model	Df	Chi-sq	Chi-sq Difference	Df Difference	p-Value	CFI Difference	TLI Difference	RMSEA Difference	SRMR Difference
Unconstrained	44	131.810	-	-	-	-	-	-	-
Constrained	70	177.990	46.180	26	0.008 **	0.009	−0.019	0.009	−0.008

Signif. codes: "**" 0.01.

The arrows in the following Figure 5 show respectively the significant association identified among the Italian frontline (see Figure 5A) and non-frontline HCWs (see Figure 5B). Asterisks indicate the level of significance of the estimated effects. Just by looking at the two figures, it is possible to notice how the structure of the relations among the variables differs noticeably in the two groups of HCWs and is more complex in the non-frontline one.

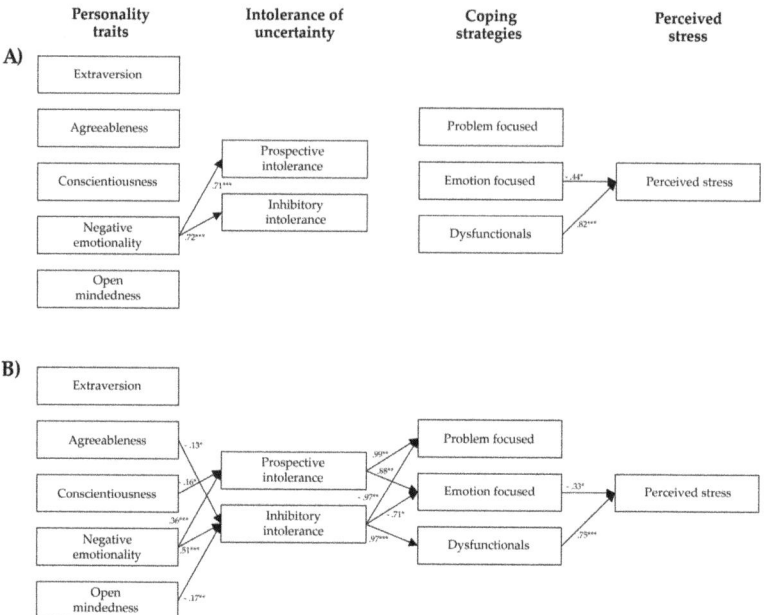

Figure 5. Structure of relations in the: (**A**) Frontline group of Italian HCWs; (**B**) non-frontline group of Italian HCWs. Signif. codes: 0 "***" 0.001, "**" 0.01, "*" 0.05, "." 0.1.

The analysis revealed significant differences in the structure of the associations between the two groups of HCWs, concerning specifically the relations between:

(a) Personality traits and Intolerance of uncertainty. While neuroticism was positively related to inhibitory and prospective intolerance of uncertainty (i.e., the more neuroticism the more intolerance of uncertainty both prospective and inhibitory) in both groups, other significant relations were found exclusively in the non-frontline HCWs. Specifically: conscientiousness was negatively related to prospective intolerance of uncertainty (i.e., the more conscientiousness, the less prospective intolerance of uncertainty. In other words, the more organized, productive, and responsible HCWs are, the less they are engaged in information-seeking to increase certainty), while agreeableness and open mindedness were negatively related to the inhibitory intolerance of uncertainty (i.e., the more agreeableness and open mindedness, the less inhibitory intolerance of uncertainty. In other words, the more confident, and intellectually creative and curious HCWs are, the less they seem to be paralyzed by uncertainty). These results seem to suggest that personality traits of frontline HCWs have a poor influence on levels of intolerance to uncertainty, except for the negative emotionality, which seems to act analogously in both HCWs' groups.

(b) Intolerance of uncertainty and Coping strategies. No significant relation was found in the frontline group of HCWs. Vice versa, in the non-frontline one, while prospective intolerance of uncertainty was positively related to problem and emotion focused coping strategies (i.e., the more prospective intolerance of uncertainty, the more problem and emotion focused coping strategies), inhibitory intolerance of uncertainty was negatively related both to problem and emotion-focused coping (i.e., the more inhibitory intolerance of uncertainty, the less problem and emotion focused coping strategies), and positively related to dysfunctional coping ones (i.e., the more inhibitory intolerance of uncertainty, the more dysfunctional coping strategies).

Regarding the relation between coping strategies and stress no difference was identified between the two groups. In both of them, emotionally focused coping was negatively related with perceived stress (i.e., the more emotion focused strategies, the less stress), whereas the dysfunctional one was positively correlated with stress (i.e., the more dysfunctional strategies, the more stress).

4. Discussion and Conclusions

COVID-19 was (and is) an arduous challenge for HCWs all over the world, but especially for those working in the areas characterized by a rapid spread of the virus, which caused, specifically during the first waves, high numbers of hospitalizations (in intensive care units) and deaths, such as in Italy [22].

Many research studies, focused on the impacts of COVID-19 on mental health [98], have revealed that HCWs, involved in fronting this pandemic as those engaged during the past ones [14–16], were at particular risk of developing severe mental symptoms due to the very demanding [24], uncertain [44], and stressful situation. Nevertheless, it is reasonable to assume that such psychological outcomes are also due to more specific contextual conditions (first of all, as argued above, having worked on the frontline or not), as well as to individual differences in personality traits, ability to tolerate uncertainty and to cope with it. Thus, the main aim of the present paper was to investigate, in a sample of 682 Italian doctors and nurses, whether specific job conditions, i.e., having worked in a dedicated COVID ward (280) or not (402) during the first wave of the pandemic in Italy, would have determined differences in the associations (i.e., in the structure of relations) between personality traits, intolerance to uncertainty, coping strategies, and perceived stress.

In line with our expectations, the analysis (LMMs) did not reveal significant differences between the two groups of Italian HCWs with regard to personality traits, intolerance of uncertainty, and coping strategies. In other words, the two groups of HCWs appear to be homogeneous not only in terms of dispositional traits, but also in terms of coping strategies adopted to face the situation, at least in the first phases of the pandemic. Conscientiousness and high levels of prospective intolerance of uncertainty seem to characterize our sample of HCWs. Both the ability to be organized, responsible, and productive (typical of the conscientious personality) and to not be paralyzed by uncertainty—but on the contrary to be engaged in information seeking, which is a typical trait of the prospective intolerance of uncertainty—seem to be focal in HCWs' work. Furthermore, resorting to coping strategies mainly focused on emotions (acceptance, seeking emotional support, humor, positive reframing, religion) seems understandable in a situation such as a pandemic, which, especially in its early stages, was characterized by high levels of uncertainty and unpredictability, and which confronted health workers every day with suffering and death.

Nonetheless, the analysis (LM) revealed higher levels of perceived stress among the frontline HCWs rather than in the non-frontline. This finding is consistent with the results of previous studies on both past epidemics [99] and the COVID-19 pandemic [17]. Specifically, during the outbreak in 2020, both Italian [100,101] and Chinese [21] frontline HCWs reported high levels of perceived stress and were more exposed to psychological burden than second line HCWs in terms of anxiety, depression, insomnia, and distress [25]. Moreover, this data seem to be understandable in the light of the increased risks faced by the frontline HCWs.

Multi-group path-analysis based on the lavaan R-software package was used and the results mainly confirmed our hypotheses, revealing for the two groups of Italian HCWs different models of associations among the variables taken into account (see Figure 5A,B). Specifically, the analysis revealed more complex associations in the non-frontline HCWs' group. This could be due to the greater heterogeneity of this group of healthcare professionals who, unlike the group who worked in dedicated COVID wards, continued to work in different types of wards (which are characterized per se by an intrinsic diversity).

Specifically, significant differences were found between frontline and non-frontline Italian HCWs concerning the associations between: personality traits and intolerance of uncertainty; intolerance of uncertainty and coping strategies.

As for the associations between personality traits and intolerance of uncertainty, among the non-frontline HCWs, high levels of conscientiousness are negatively related to prospective intolerance of uncertainty. In other words, the more they are conscientious (i.e., able from an organizational, productive, and responsible point of view), the less they show need and desire for predictability and active engagement in increasing their certainty. High levels of agreeableness and open-mindedness are, instead, in the same group, negatively related with inhibitory intolerance of uncertainty. In other words, the more individuals are agreeable (i.e., confident and compassionate) and open-minded (i.e., curious and open to the unexpected events), the less they seem to be paralyzed by inhibitory uncertainty. Vice versa, among the frontline HCWs, personality traits seem to have had a poor influence on intolerance of uncertainty, except for neuroticism, that seems to act similarly in both groups of HCWs by increasing both the prospective and inhibitory intolerance of uncertainty.

As for the associations between intolerance of uncertainty and coping strategies, no significant relationship has been identified among the frontline HCWs. It is as if knowing with certainty dealing with infected people reduces the effect of the intolerance of uncertainty on coping strategies. On the contrary, among the non-frontline HCWs, prospective intolerance of uncertainty is positively linked with problem and emotion-focused coping strategies. In other words, HCWs with high levels of prospective intolerance of uncertainty resort to problem and emotion-focused strategies in facing the situation, i.e., acting in order to reduce uncertainty. In this sense, prospective uncertainty seems to be predictive of greater use of functional coping strategies among health professionals. Vice versa, inhibitory intolerance of uncertainty is negatively related to problem and emotion-focused coping strategies (in line with its paralyzing traits) and positively related with dysfunctional coping strategies (in line with its avoidance characteristics). In other words, higher levels of inhibitory intolerance of uncertainty seem to be predictive of greater recourse to dysfunctional coping strategies. In this sense, inhibitory intolerance of uncertainty seems to have a more negative impact on HCWs' ability to cope with stressful situations rather than the prospective one.

Interesting similarities were found instead between the two groups of HCWs regarding the role of negative emotionality (neuroticism) in affecting intolerance of uncertainty, and concerning the association between coping strategies and perceived stress.

The finding according to which negative emotionality (neuroticism) affects intolerance of uncertainty is in line with the results of much research, mainly concerning general population samples [49,59,102,103], also during the pandemic [104], according to which "poor emotional regulation skills contribute to intolerance to uncertainty" [105] (p. 4). Irrespective of having worked on the frontline or not, Italian HCWs with high levels of neuroticism also showed high levels of intolerance of uncertainty (both prospective and inhibitory). In other words, neuroticism seems to be predictive of high levels of intolerance of uncertainty also among healthcare professionals irrespective of their being frontline or not.

As for the association between coping strategies and perceived stress, in both groups, resorting to emotion-focused coping strategies (acceptance, seeking emotional support, humor, positive reframing, religion) was negatively related to perceived stress, whereas the dysfunctional one was positively linked to stress. The first association we identified, according to which emotion-focused coping strategies are linked to lower level of perceived stress, thus functioning as a protective factor against negative psychological outcomes, is consistent with the results of many other studies on the general population during COVID-19 [106], as well as on HCWs before COVID-19 [107–109] and during it [110,111]. Similarly, also the second association we identified, according to which, on the contrary, dysfunctional coping strategies (behavioral disengagement, denial, self-blame, self-distraction, substance use) are linked to higher levels of perceived stress, is consistent with the results of many other studies [79,100,110], as well as in line with our expectations. Furthermore, consistently with the results of other works on Italian HCWs employed in facing COVID-19 during the first months of its spread [101,112–114], we did not find positive associations between problem-focused coping strategies and stress reduction in both groups of HCWs. Analogously to the results of these studies [101,112–114], our findings revealed that, problem-focused coping strategies were not effective in the reduction of HCWs' perceived stress during the first wave of the pandemic (that was the period the respondents of our questionnaire referred to) probably due to the "lack of scientific knowledge about the therapeutic and treatment procedures effective for COVID-19" [114] (p. 3). In other words, the insufficient knowledge and the wide-spread uncertainty about the effective procedures to apply in order to prevent the spread of the virus and to treat infected people, seem to have made it difficult for health professionals to resort to problem-focused coping as strategies for stress reduction.

There are some limitations to the current research that should be considered. The first one concerns methodology: the research used self-report measures (although exclusively validated scales has been utilized, they can lead to potential bias related to social desirability), involved a non-probabilistic sample and it was a cross-sectional study. Moreover, although information has been collected on doctors and nurses, the level of severity of the patients with whom the participants had been in contact has not been specified. Furthermore, other significant variables such as years of service (seniority), age, medical specializations, gender, etc., have not been taken into account. Finally, doctors and nurses were not randomly assigned to workplaces. In addition, we did not evaluate the role played by reasoning processes, i.e., by cognitive strategies used by HCWs to reach decisions. While non-frontline HCWs (who generally did not have to deal with virus-related emergencies) probably have had more time to process information, to evaluate possible alternatives, and to make decisions, frontline HCWs more likely have had less time to think, to consider alternatives, and to assume decisions. This may have led the frontline HCWs to resort more frequently to shortcuts in thinking (heuristics) [115,116], which may have had some influence on the associations between the variables we examined, perhaps even inhibiting or reducing the strength of dispositional traits and the associations between them. Nonetheless, since we did not take into consideration reasoning processes, their possible impact remains a supposition, which deserves to be explored in future research.

Future studies might also take into account how the socio-demographic and work-related variables impact stress, as well as other psychological outcomes, among HCWs. Furthermore, it would also be interesting to investigate HCWs' point of views, i.e., to analyze not only their responses to the items of validated scales (using quantitative methods), but also to analyze (using qualitative methods), their open-ended responses and/or interviews. Regarding this last point, our research team is qualitatively analyzing a sample of responses given to the last open-ended question of our questionnaire, which aimed to know if and how the experience of working during the pandemic had an emotional impact on HCWs (see Section 2.1). It would have been interesting also to repeat the survey after the second wave of the virus outbreak to test if new knowledge concerning the virus spread and its cure had influenced the use of coping strategies and the levels of perceived stress among Italian HCWs, and if so, how.

Despite the limitations, the results of the current study might be useful for planning and adopting preventing approaches to reduce HCWs' stress burden during a health emergency. The inability to tolerate uncertainty or the use of dysfunctional coping strategies, in fact, not only lead to negative outcomes for HCWs, but may also have an impact on patients and healthcare systems. The planning of training courses aimed to provide HCWs with skillsets they can use to cope with uncertain and stressful situations (such as that related to the COVID-19 pandemic) might be effective not only in reducing and controlling perceived stress (thus improving their mental wellbeing), but also in improving HCWs' effectiveness, and, thus have positive impacts on patients' health and on reducing costs for healthcare systems. Effective interventions should be designed to fit the specific traits of HCWs at the forefront. Health professionals who are better equipped (in psychological terms) to cope with uncertain and stressful situations would undoubtedly lead to improve the quality of care.

Author Contributions: Conceptualization, R.B. (Ramona Bongelli), C.C., A.F., M.M., I.R., A.B. and R.B. (Roberto Burro); methodology, R.B. (Roberto Burro); formal analysis, R.B. (Ramona Bongelli), A.F. and R.B. (Roberto Burro); data curation, R.B. (Ramona Bongelli), C.C., A.F., M.M., I.R., A.B. and R.B. (Roberto Burro); writing—original draft preparation, R.B. (Ramona Bongelli); writing—review and editing, R.B. (Ramona Bongelli), C.C., A.F., M.M., I.R., A.B. and R.B. (Roberto Burro); visualization, R.B. (Roberto Burro); supervision, R.B. (Ramona Bongelli). All authors have read and agreed to the published version of the manuscript.

Funding: This research received no external funding.

Institutional Review Board Statement: The study was conducted according to the guidelines of the Declaration of Helsinki, and approved by PhD meeting curriculum in Psychology, Communication, and Social Sciences, (University of Macerata. Protocol code n. 19435, 3 August 2020).

Informed Consent Statement: Informed consent was obtained from all the participants involved in the study.

Data Availability Statement: All relevant data presented in the study are included in the article. The datasets analyzed are available from the corresponding author on reasonable request.

Acknowledgments: We would like to thank professional orders and associations, as well as each doctor and nurse who compiled the questionnaire.

Conflicts of Interest: The authors declare no conflict of interest.

References

1. Wang, H.; Xia, Q.; Xiong, Z.; Li, Z.; Xiang, W.; Yuan, Y.; Liu, Y.; Li, Z. The psychological distress and coping styles in the early stages of the 2019 coronavirus disease (COVID-19) epidemic in the general mainland Chinese population: A web-based survey. *PLoS ONE* **2020**, *15*, e0233410. [CrossRef]
2. Shi, L.; Lu, Z.A.; Que, J.Y.; Huang, X.L.; Liu, L.; Ran, M.S.; Gong, Y.M.; Yuan, K.; Yan, W.; Sun, Y.K.; et al. Prevalence of and risk factors associated with mental health symptoms among the general population in China during the coronavirus disease 2019 pandemic. *JAMA Netw. Open* **2020**, *3*, e2014053. [CrossRef] [PubMed]
3. Moccia, L.; Janiri, D.; Pepe, M.; Dattoli, L.; Molinaro, M.; De Martin, V.; Chieffo, D.; Janiri, L.; Fiorillo, A.; Sani, G.; et al. Affective temperament, attachment style, and the psychological impact of the COVID-19 outbreak: An early report on the Italian general population. *Brain Behav. Immun.* **2020**, *87*, 75–79. [CrossRef]
4. Rossi, R.; Socci, V.; Talevi, D.; Mensi, S.; Niolu, C.; Pacitti, F.; Di Marco, A.; Rossi, A.; Siracusano, A.; Di Lorenzo, G. COVID-19 pandemic and lockdown measures impact on mental health among the general population in Italy. *Front. Psychiatry* **2020**, *11*, 79. [CrossRef] [PubMed]
5. Lanciano, T.; Graziano, G.; Curci, A.; Costadura, S.; Monaco, A. Risk perceptions and psychological effects during the italian COVID-19 emergency. *Front. Psychiatry* **2020**, *11*, 2434. [CrossRef] [PubMed]
6. Cullen, W.; Gulati, G.; Kelly, B.D. Mental health in the Covid-19 pandemic. *QJM* **2020**, *113*, 311–312. [CrossRef]
7. Luo, M.; Guo, L.; Yu, M.; Wang, H. The psychological and mental impact of coronavirus disease 2019 (COVID-19) on medical staff and general public—A systematic review and meta-analysis. *Psychiatry Res.* **2020**, *291*, 113190. [CrossRef] [PubMed]
8. Yao, H.; Chen, J.H.; Xu, Y.F. Patients with mental health disorders in the COVID-19 epidemic. *Lancet Psychiatry* **2020**, *7*, e21. [CrossRef]
9. Hao, F.; Tan, W.; Jiang, L.; Zhang, L.; Zhao, X.; Zou, Y.; Hu, Y.; Luo, X.; Jiang, X.; McIntyre, R.S.; et al. Do psychiatric patients experience more psychiatric symptoms during COVID-19 pandemic and lockdown? A case-control study with service and research implications for immunopsychiatry. *Brain Behav. Immun.* **2020**, *87*, 100–106. [CrossRef] [PubMed]
10. Al-Quteimat, O.M.; Amer, A.M. The impact of the COVID-19 pandemic on cancer patients. *Am. J. Clin. Oncol.* **2020**. [CrossRef] [PubMed]
11. Romito, F.; Dellino, M.; Loseto, G.; Opinto, G.; Silvestris, E.; Cormio, C.; Guarini, A.; Minoia, C. Psychological Distress in Outpatients With Lymphoma During the COVID-19 Pandemic. *Front. Oncol.* **2020**, *10*, 1270. [CrossRef] [PubMed]
12. Bargon, C.; Batenburg, M.; van Stam, L.; van der Molen, D.M.; van Dam, I.; van der Leij, F.; Baas, I.; Ernst, M.; Maarse, W.; Vermulst, N.; et al. The impact of the COVID-19 pandemic on quality of life, physical and psychosocial wellbeing in breast cancer patients—A prospective, multicenter cohort study. *Eur. J. Cancer* **2020**, *138*, S17. [CrossRef]
13. Chan, C.; Oey, N.E.; Tan, E.K. Mental health of scientists in the time of COVID-19. *Brain Behav. Immun.* **2020**, *88*, 956. [CrossRef] [PubMed]
14. Chong, M.Y.; Wang, W.C.; Hsieh, W.C.; Lee, C.Y.; Chiu, N.M.; Yeh, W.C.; Huang, T.L.; Wen, J.H.; Chen, C.L. Psychological impact of severe acute respiratory syndrome on health workers in a tertiary hospital. *Br. J. Psychiatry* **2004**, *185*, 127–133. [CrossRef]
15. Lee, A.M.; Wong, J.G.; McAlonan, G.M.; Cheung, V.; Cheung, C.; Sham, P.C.; Chu, C.M.; Wong, P.C.; Tsang, K.; Chua, S.E. Stress and psychological distress among SARS survivors 1 year after the outbreak. *Can. J. Psychiatry* **2007**, *52*, 233–240. [CrossRef]

16. Wu, P.; Fang, Y.; Guan, Z.; Fan, B.; Kong, J.; Yao, Z.; Liu, X.; Fuller, C.J.; Susser, E.; Lu, J.; et al. The psychological impact of the SARS epidemic on hospital employees in China: Exposure, risk perception, and altruistic acceptance of risk. *Can. J. Psychiatry* **2009**, *54*, 302–311. [CrossRef]
17. Cabarkapa, S.; Nadjidai, S.E.; Murgier, J.; Ng, C.H. The psychological impact of COVID-19 and other viral epidemics on frontline healthcare workers and ways to address it: A rapid systematic review. *Brain Behav. Immun. Health* **2020**, 100144. [CrossRef]
18. Ahn, M.H.; Shin, Y.W.; Kim, J.H.; Kim, H.J.; Lee, K.U.; Chung, S. High Work-related Stress and Anxiety Response to COVID-19 among Healthcare Workers in South Korea. *SAVE Study* **2020**. [CrossRef]
19. Barello, S.; Palamenghi, L.; Graffigna, G. Burnout and somatic symptoms among frontline healthcare professionals at the peak of the Italian COVID-19 pandemic. *Psychiatry Res.* **2020**, *290*, 113129. [CrossRef] [PubMed]
20. Ricci-Cabello, I.; Meneses-Echavez, J.F.; Serrano-Ripoll, M.J.; Fraile-Navarro, D.; Fiol-Roque, M.A.; Moreno, G.P.; Castro, A.; Ruiz-Pérez, I.; Campos, R.Z.; Gonçalves-Bradley, D. Impact of viral epidemic outbreaks on mental health of healthcare workers: A rapid systematic review and meta-analysis. *J. Affect. Disord.* **2020**, *277*, 347–357. [CrossRef]
21. Du, J.; Dong, L.; Wang, T.; Yuan, C.; Fu, R.; Zhang, L.; Bo, L.; Zhang, M.; Yin, Y.; Qin, J.; et al. Psychological symptoms among frontline healthcare workers during COVID-19 outbreak in Wuhan. *Gen. Hosp. Psychiatry* **2020**, *67*, 144–145. [CrossRef]
22. Giusti, E.M.; Pedroli, E.; D'Aniello, G.E.; Badiale, C.S.; Pietrabissa, G.; Manna, G.; Badiale, M.S.; Riva, G.; Castelnuovo, G.; Molinari, E. The psychological impact of the COVID-19 outbreak on health professionals: A cross-sectional study. *Front. Psychol.* **2020**, *11*, 1684. [CrossRef]
23. Guo, J.; Liao, L.; Wang, B.; Li, X.; Guo, L.; Tong, Z.; Guan, Q.; Zhou, M.; Wu, Y.; Zhang, J.; et al. Psychological effects of COVID-19 on hospital staff: A national cross-sectional survey in mainland China. *Vasc. Investig. Ther.* **2021**, *4*, 6–11. Available online: https://www.vitonline.org/article.asp?issn=2589-9686;year=2021;volume=4;issue=1;spage=6;epage=11;aulast=Guo (accessed on 23 July 2021). [CrossRef]
24. Ho, C.S.; Chee, C.; Ho, R. Mental health strategies to combat the psychological impact of coronavirus disease 2019 (COVID-19) beyond paranoia and panic. *Ann. Acad. Med. Singap.* **2020**, *49*, 1–6. Available online: http://www.anmm.org.mx/descargas/Ann-Acad-Med-Singapore.pdf (accessed on 18 August 2021). [CrossRef]
25. Lai, J.; Ma, S.; Wang, Y.; Cai, Z.; Hu, J.; Wei, N.; Wu, J.; Du, H.; Chen, T.; Li, R.; et al. Factors associated with mental health outcomes among health care workers exposed to coronavirus disease 2019. *JAMA Netw. Open* **2020**, *3*, e203976. [CrossRef] [PubMed]
26. Lam, S.C.; Arora, T.; Grey, I.; Suen, L.K.P.; Huang, E.Y.Z.; Li, D.; Lam, K.B.H. Perceived risk and protection from infection and depressive symptoms among healthcare workers in mainland China and Hong Kong during COVID-19. *Front. Psychiatry* **2020**, *11*, 686. [CrossRef] [PubMed]
27. Magnavita, N.; Tripepi, G.; Di Prinzio, R.R. Symptoms in health care workers during the covid-19 epidemic. A cross-sectional survey. *Int. J. Environ. Res. Public Health* **2020**, *17*, 5218. [CrossRef]
28. Pappa, S.; Ntella, V.; Giannakas, T.; Giannakoulis, V.G.; Papoutsi, E.; Katsaounou, P. Prevalence of depression, anxiety, and insomnia among healthcare workers during the COVID-19 pandemic: A systematic review and meta-analysis. *Brain Behav. Immun.* **2020**, *88*, 901–907. [CrossRef]
29. Preti, E.; Di Mattei, V.; Perego, G.; Ferrari, F.; Mazzetti, M.; Taranto, P.; Di Pierro, R.; Madeddu, F.; Calati, R. The psychological impact of epidemic and pandemic outbreaks on healthcare workers: Rapid review of the evidence. *Curr. Psychiatry Rep.* **2020**, *22*, 1–22. [CrossRef] [PubMed]
30. Rossi, R.; Socci, V.; Pacitti, F.; Di Lorenzo, G.; Di Marco, A.; Siracusano, A.; Rossi, A. Mental health outcomes among frontline and second-line health care workers during the coronavirus disease 2019 (COVID-19) pandemic in Italy. *JAMA Netw. Open* **2020**, *3*, e2010185. [CrossRef] [PubMed]
31. Song, X.; Ni, C.; Cai, W.; Hou, T.; Lian, B.; Chen, A.; Yin, Q.; Deng, G.; Li, H. Psychological Status of Health Care Workers during the Outbreak of Coronavirus Disease in China: A Cross-Sectional Study. 2020. Available online: https://europepmc.org/api/fulltextRepo?pprId=PPR121860&type=FILE&fileName=EMS99045-pdf.pdf&mimeType=application/pdf (accessed on 23 July 2021). [CrossRef]
32. Spoorthy, M.S.; Pratapa, S.K.; Mahant, S. Mental health problems faced by healthcare workers due to the COVID-19 pandemic–A review. *Asian J. Psychiatry* **2020**, *51*, 102119. [CrossRef]
33. Talevi, D.; Socci, V.; Carai, M.; Carnaghi, G.; Faleri, S.; Trebbi, E.; Di Bernardo, A.; Capelli, F.; Pacitti, F. Mental health outcomes of the CoViD-19 pandemic. *Riv. Psichiatry* **2020**, *55*, 137–144. [CrossRef]
34. Vagni, M.; Maiorano, T.; Giostra, V.; Pajardi, D. Hardiness, stress and secondary trauma in italian healthcare and emergency workers during the COVID-19 pandemic. *Sustainability* **2020**, *12*, 5592. [CrossRef]
35. Zhang, W.R.; Wang, K.; Yin, L.; Zhao, W.F.; Xue, Q.; Peng, M.; Min, B.; Tian, Q.; Leng, H.; Du, J.; et al. Mental health and psychosocial problems of medical health workers during the COVID-19 epidemic in China. *Psychother. Psychosom.* **2020**, *89*, 242–250. [CrossRef]
36. Zhu, Z.; Xu, S.; Wang, H.; Liu, Z.; Wu, J.; Li, G.; Miao, J.; Zhang, C.; Yang, Y.; Sun, W.; et al. COVID-19 in Wuhan: Sociodemographic characteristics and hospital support measures associated with the immediate psychological impact on healthcare workers. *EClinicalMedicine* **2020**, *24*, 100443. [CrossRef] [PubMed]

37. Rapisarda, F.; Vallarino, M.; Cavallini, E.; Barbato, A.; Brousseau-Paradis, C.; De Benedictis, L.; Lesage, A. The early impact of the Covid-19 emergency on mental health workers: A survey in Lombardy, Italy. *Int. J. Environ. Res. Public Health* **2020**, *17*, 8615. [CrossRef] [PubMed]
38. Marton, G.; Vergani, L.; Mazzocco, K.; Garassino, M.C.; Pravettoni, G. 2020s heroes are not fearless: The impact of the COVID-19 pandemic on wellbeing and emotions of italian health care workers during Italy Phase 1. *Front. Psychol.* **2020**, *11*, 2781. [CrossRef]
39. Carmassi, C.; Foghi, C.; Dell'Oste, V.; Cordone, A.; Bertelloni, C.A.; Bui, E.; Dell'Osso, L. PTSD symptoms in Healthcare Workers facing the three Coronavirus outbreaks: What can we expect after the COVID-19 pandemic. *Psychiatry Res.* **2020**, *292*, 113312. [CrossRef]
40. Yin, Q.; Sun, Z.; Liu, T.; Ni, X.; Deng, X.; Jia, D.; Shang, Z.; Zhou, Y.; Liu, W. Posttraumatic stress symptoms of health care workers during the corona virus disease 2019 (COVID-19). *Clin. Psychol. Psychother.* **2020**, *27*, 384–395. [CrossRef]
41. Gupta, S.; Sahoo, S. Pandemic and mental health of the front-line healthcare workers: A review and implications in the Indian context amidst COVID-19. *Gen. Psychiatry* **2020**, *33*, e100284. [CrossRef]
42. Lazarus, R.S.; Cohen, J.B. Environmental Stress. In *Human Behavior and Environment*; Altman, I., Wohlwill, J.F., Eds.; Springer: Boston, MA, USA, 1977; pp. 89–127.
43. Rutter, H.; Wolpert, M.; Greenhalgh, T. Managing uncertainty in the covid-19 era. *BMJ* **2020**, *370*. [CrossRef]
44. Taylor, S. *The Psychology of Pandemics: Preparing for the Next Global Outbreak of Infectious Disease*; Cambridge Scholars Publishing: Newcastle, UK, 2019.
45. Di Trani, M.; Mariani, R.; Ferri, R.; De Berardinis, D.; Frigo, M.G. From resilience to burnout in healthcare workers during the COVID-19 emergency: The role of the ability to tolerate uncertainty. *Front. Psychol.* **2021**, *12*, 987. [CrossRef]
46. Carleton, R.N. The intolerance of uncertainty construct in the context of anxiety disorders: Theoretical and practical perspectives. *Expert Rev. Neurother.* **2012**, *12*, 937–947. [CrossRef] [PubMed]
47. Fergus, T.A. A comparison of three self-report measures of intolerance of uncertainty: An examination of structure and incremental explanatory power in a community sample. *Psychol. Assesment* **2013**, *25*, 1322–1331. [CrossRef]
48. Fergus, T.A.; Bardeen, J.R. Anxiety sensitivity and intolerance of uncertainty: Evidence of incremental specificity in relation to health anxiety. *Personal. Individ. Differ.* **2013**, *55*, 640–644. [CrossRef]
49. McEvoy, P.M.; Mahoney, A.E. Achieving certainty about the structure of intolerance of uncertainty in a treatment-seeking sample with anxiety and depression. *J. Anxiety Disord.* **2011**, *25*, 112–122. [CrossRef] [PubMed]
50. McCann, S.J.H. Emotional health and the Big Five personality factors at the American state level. *J. Happiness Stud.* **2011**, *12*, 547–560. [CrossRef]
51. Asmundson, G.J.; Taylor, S. Coronaphobia: Fear and the 2019-nCoV outbreak. *J. Anxiety Disord.* **2020**, *70*, 102196. [CrossRef] [PubMed]
52. Bakioğlu, F.; Korkmaz, O.; Ercan, H. Fear of COVID-19 and positivity: Mediating role of intolerance of uncertainty, depression, anxiety, and stress. *Int. J. Ment. Health Addict* **2020**, *28*, 1–14. [CrossRef]
53. Gica, S.; Kavakli, M.; Durduran, Y.; Ak, M. The Effect of COVID-19 Pandemic on psychosomatic complaints and investigation of the mediating role of intolerance to uncertainty, biological rhythm changes and perceived COVID-19 threat in this relationship: A web-based community survey. *Psychiatry Clin. Psych.* **2020**, *30*, 89–96. [CrossRef]
54. Satici, B.; Saricali, M.; Satici, S.A.; Griffiths, M.D. Intolerance of uncertainty and mental wellbeing: Serial mediation by rumination and fear of COVID-19. *Int. J. Ment. Health Addict* **2020**, 1–12. [CrossRef]
55. Voitsidis, P.; Gliatas, I.; Bairachtari, V.; Papadopoulou, K.; Papageorgiou, G.; Parlapani, E.; Syngelakis, M.; Holeva, V.; Diakogiannis, I. Insomnia during the COVID-19 pandemic in a Greek population. *Psychiatry Res.* **2020**, *289*, 113076. [CrossRef]
56. Aksoy, Y.E.; Koçak, V. Psychological effects of nurses and midwives due to COVID-19 outbreak: The case of Turkey. *Arch. Psychiatry Nurs.* **2020**, *34*, 427–433. [CrossRef] [PubMed]
57. McKay, D.; Minaya, C.; Storch, E.A. Conducting exposure and response prevention treatment for contamination fears during COVID-19: The behavioral immune system impact on clinician approaches to treatment. *J. Anxiety Disord.* **2020**, *74*, 102270. [CrossRef]
58. Tull, M.T.; Barbano, A.C.; Scamaldo, K.M.; Richmond, J.R.; Edmonds, K.A.; Rose, J.P.; Gratz, K.L. The prospective influence of COVID-19 affective risk assessments and intolerance of uncertainty on later dimensions of health anxiety. *J. Anxiety Disord.* **2020**, *75*, 102290. [CrossRef]
59. McEvoy, P.M.; Mahoney, A.E. Intolerance of uncertainty and negative metacognitive beliefs as transdiagnostic mediators of repetitive negative thinking in a clinical sample with anxiety disorders. *J. Anxiety Disord.* **2013**, *27*, 216–224. [CrossRef] [PubMed]
60. Lazarus, R.S.; Folkman, S. *Stress, Appraisal, and Coping*; Springer Publishing Company: New York, NY, USA, 1984.
61. Lazarus, R.S. *Psychological Stress and the Coping Process*; McGraw-Hill: New York, NY, USA, 1996.
62. Monzani, D.; Steca, P.; Greco, A.; D'Addario, M.; Cappelletti, E.; Pancani, L. The situational version of the Brief COPE: Dimensionality and relationships with goal-related variables. *Eur. J. Psychol.* **2015**, *11*, 295–310. [CrossRef] [PubMed]
63. Mache, S. Coping with job stress by hospital doctors: A comparative study. *Wiener Medizinische Wochenschrift* **2012**, *162*, 440–447. [CrossRef]
64. Folkman, S.; Lazarus, R.S. An analysis of coping in a middle-aged community sample. *J. Health Soc. Behav.* **1980**, *21*, 219–239. [CrossRef]

65. Carver, C.S.; Scheier, M.F.; Weintraub, J.K. Assessing coping strategies: A theoretically based approach. *J. Personal. Soc. Psychol.* **1989**, *56*, 267–283. [CrossRef]
66. Carver, C.S. You want to measure coping but your protocol's too long: Consider the brief cope. *Int. J. Behav. Med.* **1997**, *4*, 92. [CrossRef] [PubMed]
67. Carver, C.S.; Scheier, M.F. *On the Self-Regulation of Behavior*; Cambridge University Press: New York, NY, USA, 1998.
68. Meyer, B. Coping with severe mental illness: Relations of the Brief COPE with symptoms, functioning, and well-being. *J. Psychopathol. Behav.* **2001**, *23*, 265–277. [CrossRef]
69. Connor-Smith, J.K.; Flachsbart, C. Relations between personality and coping: A meta-analysis. *J. Personal. Soc. Psychol.* **2007**, *93*, 1080–1107. [CrossRef] [PubMed]
70. Leandro, P.G.; Castillo, M.D. Coping with stress and its relationship with personality dimensions, anxiety, and depression. *Procedia Soc. Behav. Sci.* **2010**, *5*, 1562–1573. [CrossRef]
71. Afshar, H.; Roohafza, H.R.; Keshteli, A.H.; Mazaheri, M.; Feizi, A.; Adibi, P. The association of personality traits and coping styles according to stress level. *J. Res. Med. Sci.* **2015**, *20*, 353–358. Available online: https://www.ncbi.nlm.nih.gov/pmc/articles/PMC4468450/ (accessed on 22 August 2021). [PubMed]
72. Taylor, S.; Landry, C.A.; Paluszek, M.M.; Fergus, T.A.; McKay, D.; Asmund, G. COVID stress syndrome: Concept, structure, and correlates. *Depress. Anxiety* **2020**, *37*, 706–714. [CrossRef]
73. Munawar, K.; Choudhry, F.R. Exploring stress coping strategies of frontline emergency health workers dealing covid-19 in Pakistan: A qualitative inquiry. *Am. J. Infect. Control* **2020**. Available online: https://www.ajicjournal.org/article/S0196-6553(20)30638-6/fulltext#seccesectitle0001 (accessed on 27 July 2021). [CrossRef]
74. Salman, M.; Raza, M.H.; Mustafa, Z.U.; Khan, T.M.; Asif, N.; Tahir, H.; Shehzadi, N.; Hussain, K. The psychological effects of COVID-19 on frontline healthcare workers and how they are coping: A web-based, cross-sectional study from Pakistan. *medRxiv* **2020**. Available online: https://www.medrxiv.org/content/10.1101/2020.06.03.20119867v1 (accessed on 18 August 2021). [CrossRef]
75. Huang, L.; Lei, W.; Xu, F.; Liu, H.; Yu, L. Emotional responses and coping strategies in nurses and nursing students during Covid-19 outbreak: A comparative study. *PLoS ONE* **2020**, *15*, e0237303. [CrossRef]
76. Taha, S.; Matheson, K.; Cronin, T.; Anisman, H. Intolerance of uncertainty, appraisals, coping, and anxiety: The case of the 2009 H1N1 pandemic. *Br. J. Health Psych.* **2014**, *19*, 592–605. [CrossRef]
77. Rettie, H.; Daniels, J. Coping and tolerance of uncertainty: Predictors and mediators of mental health during the COVID-19 pandemic. *Am. Psychol.* **2020**, *76*, 427–437. [CrossRef]
78. Sica, C.; Latzman, R.D.; Caudek, C.; Cerea, S.; Colpizzi, I.; Caruso, M.; Giulini, P.; Bottesi, G. Facing distress in Coronavirus era: The role of maladaptive personality traits and coping strategies. *Personal. Individ. Differ.* **2021**, *177*, 110833. [CrossRef]
79. Liu, S.; Lithopoulos, A.; Zhang, C.Q.; Garcia-Barrera, M.A.; Rhodes, R.E. Personality and perceived stress during COVID-19 pandemic: Testing the mediating role of perceived threat and efficacy. *Personal. Individ. Differ.* **2021**, *168*, 110351. [CrossRef] [PubMed]
80. Soto, C.J.; John, O.P. Short and extra-short forms of the Big Five Inventory–2: The BFI-2-S and BFI-2-XS. *J. Res. Personal.* **2017**, *68*, 69–81. [CrossRef]
81. Soto, C.J.; John, O.P. The next big five inventory (BFI-2): Developing and assessing a hierarchical model with 15 facets to enhance bandwidth, fidelity, and predictive power. *J. Personal. Soc. Psychol.* **2017**, *113*, 117–143. [CrossRef]
82. Goldberg, L.R. The structure of phenotypic personality traits. *Am. Psychol.* **1993**, *48*, 26–34. [CrossRef]
83. John, O.P.; Naumann, L.P.; Soto, C.J. Paradigm shift to the integrative Big—Five trait taxonomy: History, measurement, and conceptual issues. In *Handbook of Personality: Theory and Research*, 3rd ed.; John, O.P., Robins, R.W., Pervin, L.A., Eds.; Guilford: New York, NY, USA, 2008; pp. 114–158.
84. McCrae, R.R.; Costa, P.T. The Five-Factor theory of personality. In *Handbook of Personality: Theory and Research*, 3rd ed.; John, O.P., Robins, R.W., Pervin, L.A., Eds.; Guilford: New York, NY, USA, 2008; pp. 159–181.
85. Kline, R.B. *Principles and Practice of Structural Equation modeling*, 4th ed.; Guilford: New York, NY, USA, 2016.
86. Bottesi, G.; Ghisi, M.; Novara, C.; Bertocchi, J.; Boido, M.; De Dominicis, I. Intolerance of uncertainty scale (IUS-27 e IUS-12): Due studi preliminari. *Psicoterapia Cognitiva e Comportamentale* **2015**, *21*, 345–365. Available online: https://www.researchgate.net/profile/Mark-Freeston/publication/281899656_Intolerance_of_Uncertainty_Scale_IUS-27_and_IUS-12_Two_preliminary_studies/links/584683ba08ae61f75ddb7faa/Intolerance-of-Uncertainty-Scale-IUS-27-and-IUS-12-Two-preliminary-studies.pdf (accessed on 22 August 2021).
87. Carleton, R.N.; Norton, P.J.; Asmundson, G.J.G. Fearing the unknown: A short version of the Intolerance of Uncertainty Scale. *J. Anxiety Disord.* **2007**, *21*, 105–117. [CrossRef]
88. Freeston, M.H.; Rhéaume, J.; Letarte, H.; Dugas, M.J.; Ladouceur, R. Why do people worry? *Personal. Individ. Differ.* **1994**, *17*, 791–802. [CrossRef]
89. Lauriola, M.; Mosca, O.; Carleton, R.N. Hierarchical factor structure of the intolerance of uncertainty scale short form (IUS-12) in the Italian version. *Test. Psychom. Methodol. Appl. Psychol.* **2016**, *23*, 377–394. [CrossRef]
90. Eisenberg, S.A.; Shen, B.J.; Schwarz, E.R.; Mallon, S. Avoidant coping moderates the association between anxiety and patient-rated physical functioning in heart failure patients. *J. Behav. Med.* **2012**, *35*, 253–261. [CrossRef]
91. Fossati, A. Scala per lo Stress Percepito. Available online: https://www.futuremedicalinnovation.it//wp-content/uploads/2017/10/ps_questionario_stress.pdf (accessed on 18 August 2021).

92. Cohen, S.; Kamarck, T.; Mermelstein, R. A global measure of perceived stress. *J. Health. Soc. Behav.* **1983**, *24*, 386–396. [CrossRef]
93. Cohen, S.; Williamson, G. Perceived stress in a probability sample of the United States. In *The Social Psychology of Health*; Spacapan, S., Oskamp, S., Eds.; Sage: Newbury Park, CA, USA, 1988; pp. 31–67.
94. Mondo, M.; Sechi, C.; Cabras, C. Psychometric evaluation of three versions of the Italian perceived stress scale. *Curr. Psychol.* **2019**, *40*, 1–9. [CrossRef]
95. Cohen, S. Perceives Stress Scale. Available online: https://www.northottawawellnessfoundation.org/wp-content/uploads/2018/04/PerceivedStressScale.pdf (accessed on 22 August 2021).
96. R Core Team. *R: A Language and Environment for Statistical Computing*; R Foundation for Statistical Computing: Vienna, Austria, 2021; Available online: https://www.R-project.org/ (accessed on 18 August 2021).
97. Rosseel, Y. Lavaan: An R Package for structural equation modeling. *J. Stat. Softw.* **2012**, *48*, 1–36. [CrossRef]
98. Usher, K.; Durkin, J.; Bhullar, N. The COVID-19 pandemic and mental health impacts. *Int. J. Ment. Health Nurs.* **2020**, *29*, 315–318. [CrossRef]
99. Tam, C.W.; Pang, E.P.; Lam, L.C.; Chiu, H.F. Severe acute respiratory syndrome (SARS) in Hong Kong in 2003: Stress and psychological impact among frontline healthcare workers. *Psychol. Med.* **2004**, *34*, 1197–1204. [CrossRef]
100. Trumello, C.; Bramanti, S.M.; Ballarotto, G.; Candelori, C.; Cerniglia, L.; Cimino, S.; Crudele, M.; Lombardi, L.; Pignataro, S.; Viceconti, M.L.; et al. Psychological adjustment of healthcare workers in Italy during the COVID-19 pandemic: Differences in stress, anxiety, depression, burnout, secondary trauma, and compassion satisfaction between frontline and non-frontline professionals. *Int. J. Environ. Res. Public Health* **2020**, *17*, 8358. [CrossRef]
101. Babore, A.; Lombardi, L.; Viceconti, M.L.; Pignataro, S.; Marino, V.; Crudele, M.; Candelori, C.; Bramanti, S.M.; Trumello, C. Psychological effects of the COVID-2019 pandemic: Perceived stress and coping strategies among healthcare professionals. *Psychiatry Res.* **2020**, *293*, 113366. [CrossRef]
102. McEvoy, P.M.; Mahoney, A.E. To be sure, to be sure: Intolerance of uncertainty mediates symptoms of various anxiety disorders and depression. *Behav. Ther.* **2012**, *43*, 533–545. [CrossRef]
103. Hawes, M.T.; Farrell, M.R.; Cannone, J.L.; Finsaas, M.C.; Olino, T.M.; Klein, N. Early childhood temperament predicts intolerance of uncertainty in adolescence. *J. Anxiety Disord.* **2021**, *80*, 102390. [CrossRef]
104. Taylor, S.; Fong, A.; Asmundson, G.J. Predicting the severity of symptoms of the COVID stress syndrome from personality traits: A prospective network analysis. *Front. Psychol.* **2021**, *12*, 1582. [CrossRef]
105. Ruckmani, V.S. Psychological perspective of uncertainty. In *The Opportunities of Uncertainties: Flexibility and Adaptation Needed in Current Climate*; Shahana, A.M., Sivakumar, A., Parthiban, V., Eds.; Lulu Publication: Raleigh, NC, USA, 2021; Volume 1, pp. 1–9.
106. Fluharty, M.; Bu, F.; Steptoe, A.; Fancourt, D. Coping strategies and mental health trajectories during the first 21 weeks of COVID-19 lockdown in the United Kingdom. *Soc. Sci. Med.* **2021**, *279*, 113958. [CrossRef] [PubMed]
107. Folkman, S.; Lazarus, R.S.; Gruen, R.J.; DeLongis, A. Appraisal, coping, health status, and psychological symptoms. *J. Personal. Soc. Psychol.* **1986**, *50*, 571. [CrossRef]
108. Lambert, V.; Lambert, C.; Ito, M. Workplace stressors, ways of coping and demographic characteristics as predictors of physical and mental health of Japanese hospital nurses. *Int. J. Nurs. Stud.* **2004**, *41*, 85–97. [CrossRef]
109. Laranjeira, C.A. The effects of perceived stress and ways of coping in a sample of Portuguese health workers. *J. Clin. Nurs.* **2012**, *21*, 1755–1762. [CrossRef]
110. Besirli, A.; Erden, S.C.; Atilgan, M.; Varlihan, A.; Habaci, M.F.; Yeniceri, T.; Isler, A.C.; Gumus, M.; Kizilerogu, S.; Ozturk, G.; et al. The Relationship between Anxiety and Depression Levels with Perceived Stress and Coping Strategies in Health Care Workers during the COVID-19 Pandemic. *Sisli. Etfal. Hastan. Tıp. Bul.* **2021**, *55*, 1. [CrossRef]
111. Canestrari, C.; Bongelli, R.; Fermani, A.; Riccioni, I.; Bertolazzi, A.; Muzi, M.; Burro, R. Coronavirus disease stress among italian healthcare workers: The role of coping humor. *Front. Psychol.* **2021**, *11*, 3962. [CrossRef]
112. Vagni, M.; Maiorano, T.; Giostra, V.; Pajardi, D. Coping with COVID-19: Emergency stress, secondary trauma and self-efficacy in healthcare and emergency workers in Italy. *Front. Psychol.* **2020**, *11*, 566912. [CrossRef] [PubMed]
113. Maiorano, T.; Vagni, M.; Giostra, V.; Pajardi, D. COVID-19: Risk factors and protective role of resilience and coping strategies for emergency stress and secondary trauma in medical staff and emergency workers—An online-based inquiry. *Sustainability* **2020**, *12*, 9004. [CrossRef]
114. Vagni, M.; Maiorano, T.; Giostra, V.; Pajardi, D. Protective factors against emergency stress and burnout in healthcare and emergency workers during second wave of COVID-19. *Soc. Sci.* **2021**, *10*, 178. [CrossRef]
115. Kahneman, D.; Slovic, S.P.; Slovic, P.; Tversky, A. (Eds.) *Judgment Under Uncertainty: Heuristics and Biases*; Cambridge University Press: Cambridge, UK, 1982.
116. Gigerenzer, G.; Gaissmaier, W. Heuristic decision making. *Annu. Rev. Psychol.* **2011**, *62*, 451–482. [CrossRef] [PubMed]

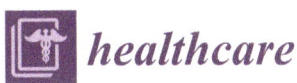

Article

Work-Related Stressors among the Healthcare Professionals in the Fever Clinic Centers for Individuals with Symptoms of COVID-19

Saad Alyahya [1,*] and Fouad AboGazalah [2]

[1] Nudge Unit, Ministry of Health, Riyadh 12628, Saudi Arabia
[2] Family Medicine, Health Holding Company, Riyadh 12584, Saudi Arabia; Fabogazalah@moh.gov.sa
* Correspondence: 11.saad.99@gmail.com; Tel.: +966-505141267

Abstract: Work-related stress can affect the quality of healthcare during the COVID-19 pandemic. This study aimed to assess the relationship between selected work-related stressors and stress levels among healthcare professionals providing preventive and curative services to people with COVID-19 symptoms in the Fever Clinics in Saudi Arabia. A systematic random sampling using an online questionnaire approach was used to select healthcare professionals in the Fever Clinics in Saudi Arabia during September 2020. Participants were asked to fill out a questionnaire including data on their sociodemographic and occupational characteristics, role conflict and ambiguity, social support, and stress. The results showed that role conflict and ambiguity were significant risk factors for stress, and social support was negatively associated with stress levels. Additionally, younger and non-Saudi healthcare professionals exhibited higher stress levels than their older and Saudi counterparts. In conclusion, role conflict, ambiguity, and social support can predict the risk of stress among healthcare professionals in the Fever Clinics in Saudi Arabia.

Keywords: stress; role conflict; role ambiguity; social support; COVID-19; Saudi Arabia

1. Introduction

Before the end of 2019, the World Health Organization (WHO) was informed of pneumonia cases discovered in Wuhan, Hubei Province, China, which was named the 2019 novel coronavirus disease (COVID-19) caused by the novel coronavirus (SARS-CoV-2) [1].

On 11 March 2020, the World Health Organization declared coronavirus (COVID-19) a pandemic, which means a global disease outbreak threatening the world [2,3] After the World Health Organization announced the pandemic, Saudi Arabia adopted response plans to contain the virus [4]. From 2 March 2020, to 2 March 2021, Saudi Arabia confirmed 377,700 cases of COVID-19 with 6500 deaths [5].

The Kingdom of Saudi Arabia has implemented many precautionary measures to prevent the spread and transmission of the SARS-CoV-2 virus, such as preventing mass gatherings, stopping school proceedings, stopping Hajj and Umrah, introducing curfews, and closing places to counter the increase in the transmission of infection [6–8]. The country has converted more than 119 health centers to receive only those infected with infection symptoms; they cover all regions and cities of the Kingdom of Saudi Arabia and receive citizens, residents, and immigrants into the country. These clinics, known as Fever Clinics, work to contain the coronavirus's spread among society members [9].

COVID-19 is the world's biggest public health threat. The severity of the disease, the lack of evidence of the effectiveness of potential therapeutic agents and the available vaccines, and the lack of presumed immunity in the population leave everyone vulnerable to infection [10,11]. Additionally, the rapid spread of COVID-19, its health implications, the wide coverage that this disease gets in the press and social media, and the horrific statistics associated with it may lead to an increase in anxiety levels and the level of adverse effects on mental health among members of society [12,13].

A number of members in the society have been affected by different psychological influences, including health care workers, who are considered one of the essential elements in protecting community members from having the virus [12,14,15]. Several studies revealed that fear of this novel coronavirus might lead to psychological issues such as stress disorders, anxiety, and depression among individuals [16]. This outbreak is not the first in the Kingdom of Saudi Arabia, since it has experienced the MERS virus epidemic before. This epidemic spread to the Middle East, affecting health workers and killing some of them, causing many psychological problems such as stress [17–19].

Stress may be affected by many variables related to the professional and social role, such as ambiguity, role conflict, and increased workload [20]. Several studies have found that workload, role ambiguity, and role conflict are factors associated with stress and that these factors degrade employee job satisfaction and performance [21–23]. Based on this, too much stress may negatively affect both the employees' and the organization's work performance.

In contrast, social support is a preventative factor against mental health problems in the workplace [24]. Social support is the care or help that a person can feel, notice, or accept from others. A high social support level can protect someone under stress [25,26]. The more social support the person has or perceives, the more control of the person's stressful situation, leading to improved outcomes associated with it [27,28].

All these factors, including role ambiguity, role conflict, work overload, and social support, may influence the level of stress among health sector workers, especially during the novel coronavirus pandemic.

Therefore, to the authors' knowledge, this study is considered the first of its kind. This study seeks to determine the relationship between the variables associated with stress, such as ambiguity and role conflict, workload, and social support, among health sector workers, specifically in health centers called Fever Clinics centers designated to receive those with symptoms of COVID-19 infection in the Kingdom of Saudi Arabia.

2. Materials and Methods

This study used data from Almansour et al., study of Work-Related Challenges among Primary Health Centers Workers during COVID-19 in Saudi Arabia [29]. The random sampling technique was used in the original national cross-sectional study. The original study aimed to explore the association between role conflict, role ambiguity, self-esteem, and social support with stress levels among HCWs in primary healthcare centers in Saudi Arabia, including regular primary health centers and Fever Clinic centers. The original study also aimed to identify the differences in stress, role conflict and ambiguity, self-esteem, and social support between employees in regular healthcare centers and Fever Clinics.

An online questionnaire was used to collect data from the participants using a multi-stage random sampling approach. The study participants were selected from the employees in the primary healthcare center of the five geographical regions of Saudi Arabia. The study participants were recruited from 20 Directorates of Health Affairs in Saudi Arabia divided into Central, Eastern, Western, Northern, and Southern regions. All the public government primary health care centers (regular or Fever Clinic centers) fall in these 20 Directorates of Health Affairs, so every primary health care center has a chance to be selected in this study. The number of regular primary healthcare centers was 2070, while the number of Fever Clinic centers was 119. In the original study, six regular health centers and two Fever Clinics centers were randomly selected from directorates in all regions. An email was sent to each employee in the selected health centers, and a reminder email was sent a week later. A link to an electronic self-administrated questionnaire was provided in the email, and it was anticipated to be completed in 10 min. The time frame for data collection was three weeks began on 27 September 2020.

The design of the present study was nonexperimental, correlational, and cross-sectional. This study aimed to understand the sample characteristics better and investigate the work-related factors (conflict, ambiguity, overload, and social support) that can contribute to stress among health care workers in the Fever Clinic centers.

2.1. Sample

The original study's target population was the various employees in the primary healthcare centers, including healthcare professionals such as nurses, physicians, pharmacists, social workers, and the administration department employees in the healthcare centers. Emails were sent inviting the employees from the randomly selected healthcare centers to take part in the study. The emails sent out saw a 69% response rate: 1378 responses were received from the 2007 emails sent out. The data collection in each health directorate was coordinated by the head of the primary healthcare center Health Affairs Directorate. The link to the self-administered electronic questionnaire was mailed to the employees by the head of the primary healthcare center. The participants were assisted by the principal investigator when they experienced any challenges with the questionnaire. The target participants also received a weekly reminder during the data collection period.

This current study has a sample size $N = 275$ of health care workers extracted from the original dataset. The current study selected only health care workers who work in the Fever Clinics centers (20% of the original sample); health care workers who work in the regular health care centers were excluded from the current study (80% of the original sample). A conducted power analysis of the currently selected sample size of $N = 275$ using G*Power software, version 3.1.9.7, showed that this sample size has around 80% power (1-Beta error) at an alpha of 0.05, with four predictors, and one criterion, to detect even a modest effect size of 0.04 [30].

2.2. Study Variables

The study had both dependent and independent variables. The study's dependent variable was stress, while there were several independent variables, including work conflict, work ambiguity, work overload, and social support.

2.2.1. Stress

Lazarus and Folkman defined stress as "a relationship with the environment that the person appraises as significant for his or her wellbeing and in which the demands tax or exceed available coping resources" [20]. Stress was measured using the Perceived Stress Scale (PSS) about events in the last month using the following items: upset because of something that happened unexpectedly; unable to control the important things in your life; nervous and "stressed"; confident about your ability to handle your personal problems; things were going your way; you could not cope with all the things that you had to do; you have been able to control irritations in your life; you were on top of things; angered because of things that were outside of your control; and difficulties were piling up so high that you could not overcome them. This scale has been used significantly in measuring the stress estimates with strong psychometric properties [31]. Cohen et al. argue that PSS is highly correlated with various scales, making it have good validity. These may include health behavior measures, smoking status, help-seeking behavior, self-reported health, and health services measures. The participants assessed the intensity to which life stressors were overwhelming and unmanageable over the previous month. They used a scale ranging from 0 (never) to 4 (very often), with a higher score referring to a higher stress level. The scale in the original study has good reliability and validity (Cronbach's alpha 0.85).

2.2.2. Work Role Conflict

Role conflict is "the extent to which one experiences incompatible work demands" [32]. This study uses the role conflict measure for workers developed by Bowling et al. to evaluate the work-role conflict among primary healthcare workers [32]. The measure has six items and provided answers ranging from 1 (strongly disagree) to 7 (strongly agree), with a higher score on the scale pointing to a higher conflict level. The scale includes the following items: in my job, I often feel like different people are "pulling me in different directions"; I have to deal with competing demands at work; my superiors often tell me to do two different things that cannot both be done; the tasks I am assigned at work rarely come into conflict with each other; the things I am told to do at work do not conflict with each other, in my job; and I am seldom placed in a situation where one job duty conflicts with other job duties. In the original study, the scale has a reliability (Chronbach's Alpha = 0.62) which is acceptable reliability [33], as well as criterion validity with the Perceived Stress Scale (r = 0.472, $p < 0.01$).

2.2.3. Work Role Ambiguity

This variable is defined as "The extent to which one is confronted with unclear work situations" [32]. The ambiguity instrument used in this study measures role ambiguity using six items measured on a 7-point Likert scale ranging from 1 (strongly disagree) to 7 (strongly agree). The scale includes the following items: I am not sure what is expected of me at work; the requirements of my job are not always clear; I often do not know what is expected of me at work; I know everything that I am expected to do at work with certainty; My job duties are clearly defined; and I know what I am required to do for most or every aspect of my job. A higher score on this scale reflects higher role ambiguity. In the original study, the scale has good reliability (Chronbach's Alpha = 0.85) and a suitable criterion validity with Perceived Stress Scale (r = 0.478, $p < 0.01$).

2.2.4. Work Overload

Work overload has been defined as the extent to which the "job performance required in a job is excessive or overload due to performance required on a job" [34]. In the original study, work overload is measured using one question. The participants were asked how many hours they work every day. Their answers are the number of working hours.

2.2.5. Social Support

The Multidimensional Scale of Perceived Social Support (MSPSS) was used for this variable. MSPSS identifies perceptions of support from three critical elements of individuals' emotional support: family, friends, and significant others; and has 12 self-administered items [35]. The scale items are: there is a special person who is around when I am in need; there is a special person with whom I can share joys and sorrows; my family really tries to help me; I get the emotional help and support I need from my family; I have a special person who is a real source of comfort to me; my friends really try to help me; I can count on my friends when things go wrong; I can talk about my problems with my family; I have friends with whom I can share my joys and sorrows; there is a special person in my life who cares about my feelings; my family is willing to help me make decisions; and I can talk about my problems with my friends. The answer choices are in the form of a 7-point Likert scale ranging from 1 (very strongly disagree) to 7 (very strongly agree), with a higher score on the scale showing higher social support. Original study found that the scale had good reliability (Cronbach's alpha 0.92) and criterion validity (r = −0.332, $p < 0.01$).

2.3. Data Analysis

This study provided descriptive analysis, including measures of central tendency and variability for the demographic characteristics. Additionally, the chi-square test was used to compare the participants' characteristics based on the stress levels (low, moderate, and high). Bivariate correlation examined individual relationships between the level of stress (criterion variable) and the predictors. Multiple regression analysis was used to identify which of the work-related factors were best predictors for stress level. Beta scores (standardized coefficients) allowed identifying those variables with the most significant contribution to informal caregivers' emotional stress.

3. Results

Table 1 provides the descriptive statistics for the demographic variables to give the respondents' background characteristics. The average age of respondents is 38.9 years, with a standard deviation of 8.12. The results show that 36 (13.1%) respondents are less than 30 years of age, 186 (67.8%) are between ages 31 and 45, and 53 (19.3%) are 46 or older. For gender, the percentage of male respondents tends to be higher than that of female, which is 154 (56%) and 121 (44%), respectively. Additionally, most of the respondents (84.7%) are married or living together, 9.5% have never been married or single, while only 3.6% had earlier been married but then divorced or separated. The great majority of the respondents, 230 (83.6%), are citizens, while only 45 (16.4%) of them are non-residents or non-citizens. Regarding their education level, most of the respondents have attained two years of college education (42.6%), followed by those with bachelor's education (36.7%), 9.5% in graduate-level, and 7.6% attaining high school education or less. Regarding the experience with primary health centers (PHCs), the majority are those with more than ten years of experience (48.4%), 28.7% of the respondents have five years or less of experience, and those with 6 to 10 years of experience are only 22.9% of the respondents.

Table 1. Demographic characteristics.

Variable	n	%	M	SD
Age			38.9	8.13
Less than 30 years	36	13.1		
31 to 45 years	186	67.6		
46 years or older	53	19.3		
Gender				
Male	154	56.0		
Female	121	44.0		
Marital Status				
Single	32	9.5		
Married	233	84.7		
Divorced	10	3.6		
Nationality				
Citizen	230	83.6		
Not citizen	45	16.4		
Education Level				
High school or less	21	7.6		
Two years college	127	46.2		
Bachelor	101	36.7		
Graduate	26	9.5		
Experience in PHCs				
5 years or less	79	28.7		
6–10 years	63	22.9		
More than 10 years	133	48.4		

Table 2 shows the Pearson Correlation coefficients between the study's independent variables (conflict, ambiguity, overload, and social support) and the dependent variable of stress. All the independent variables in the study have a positive significant correlation with stress except overload, which has a significant negative correlation. The result was: conflict ($r = 0.487$, $p < 0.01$), ambiguity ($r = 0.479$, $p < 0.01$), overload ($r = -0.332$, $p < 0.01$), and social support ($r = 0.090$, $p < 0.01$). Additionally, conflict was found significantly correlated with ambiguity ($r = 0.509$, $p < 0.01$), overload ($r = -0.206$, $p < 0.01$), and social support ($r = 0.079$, $p < 0.01$). Ambiguity exhibited significant negative correlation with overload ($r = -0.265$, $p < 0.01$) and social support ($r = -0.026$, $p < 0.01$). Finally, overload had a negative significant correlation with social support ($r = -0.013$, $p < 0.01$). These results give a clear evidence that most of the independent variables exhibited significant correlation with each other.

Table 2. Pearson Correlation between stress and the study variables.

Variable	1	2	3	4	5
Stress	1				
Conflict	0.487 **	1			
Ambiguity	0.479 **	0.509 **	1		
Overload	−0.332 **	−0.206 **	−0.265 **	1	
Social support	0.090 **	0.079 **	−0.026 **	−0.013 **	1

Note. ** Correlation is significant at the 0.01 level (2-tailed).

The study used a chi-square test to compare healthcare workers' demographics and working hours in the Fever Clinics to improve the understanding of their characteristics based on their stress level (Low, Moderate, and High). These results are presented in Table 3. The result showed a significant difference related to participants' age groups. Younger health care workers more likely to have higher stress than the other age groups. The analysis on workers' nationality showed significant differences; non-Saudi health care workers have higher stress than Saudis. Gender, marital status, and level of education did not show significant differences in their level of stress. Additionally, working hours change did not reveal any significant differences in the stress level among the Fever Clinics' health care workers.

Table 3. Demographic characteristics by stress levels.

Variables	Low Stress Mean (±SD)	Moderate Stress Mean (±SD)	High Stress Mean (±SD)	p-Value
Age				
18–35 years	21 (30.4%)	72 (43.4%)	22 (55%)	
36–45 years	29 (42%)	61 (36.7%)	17 (42.5%)	$p < 0.05$
46–60 years	19 (27.5%)	33 (19.9%)	1 (2.5%)	
Gender				
Male	23 (33.3%)	78 (47%)	20 (50%)	$p > 0.05$
Female	46 (66.7%)	88 (53%)	20 (50%)	
Nationality				
Saudi	20 (29%)	22 (13.3%)	3 (7.5%)	$p < 0.01$
Non-Saudi	49 (71%)	144 (86.7%)	37 (92.5%)	
Marital Status				
Not Married	6 (8.7%)	32 (19.3)	4 (10%)	$p > 0.05$
Married	63 (91.3%)	134 (80.7%)	36 (90%)	
Education level				
High school or less	7 (10.1%)	13 (7.8%)	1 (2.5%)	
Two years college	32 (46.4%)	76 (45.8%)	19 (47.5)	$p > 0.05$
Bachelor	23 (33.3%)	64 (38.6%)	14 (35%)	
Graduate	7 (10.1%)	13 (7.8%)	6 (15%)	
Since COVID-19 work				
More hours	40 (58%)	112 (67.5%)	26 (65%)	$p > 0.05$
Same or fewer hours	29 (42%)	54 (32.5%)	14 (35%)	

Table 4 shows multiple regression analysis results between the criterion of stress and the predictors of conflict, ambiguity, social support, and overload. The multiple regression results indicated a significant collective effect between the independent variables of conflict, ambiguity, social support, and the dependent variable of stress. The overload was dropped from the model by the SPSS and it might be dropped because of using a single item to measure the overload. According to the result, the significant predictors based on their magnitude are: (ambiguity (Beta = 327, $p < 0.001$), conflict (Beta = 313, $p < 0.001$), and social support (Beta = −0.150, $p < 0.01$)). R square = 0.36, so all of these factors together explained 36.4% of perceived stress.

Table 4. Multiple regression analysis: predictors of stress.

Variable	B	SE	β	t	p	95.0% Confidence Interval for B	
						Lower Bound	Upper Bound
Ambiguity	2.409	0.416	0.327	5.794	0.000	1.591	3.228
Conflict	0.336	0.060	0.313	5.559	0.000	0.217	0.455
Social Support	−0.091	0.030	−0.150	−3.035	0.003	−0.149	−0.032
Constant	6.416	2.687		2.388	0.018	1.127	11.706
Adjusted R^2		0.364					
F		53.31 **					

Note. ** $p < 0.01$ level (2-tailed).

4. Discussion

This study unveiled several work-related risk factors for stress among healthcare professionals managing COVID-19 in the Fever Clinics in Saudi Arabia. While role conflict and ambiguity were positively associated with stress levels, social support was inversely associated with stress levels.

Our results concurred with a recent study conducted on healthcare professionals in primary healthcare centers in Saudi Arabia during the COVID-19 time that showed high role conflict and ambiguity levels, especially among those working at the Fever Clinics. This research also showed a tight correlation between work-related stressors and stress levels [29]. Additionally, one study in the pre-COVID-19 time conducted on healthcare professionals from Italy showed that role ambiguity was a significant risk factor for emotional exhaustion and negatively affected participants' wellbeing and psychosocial competence [36].

The Minister of Health in Saudi Arabia initiated the Fever Clinics in the wake of the COVID-19 pandemic to offer preventive and curative services for people showing COVID-19 symptoms. Given the rapidly changing guidelines and protocols of COVID-19 management and the fact that the scientific knowledge on the virus is still limited, the Fever Clinics' healthcare professionals might have incomplete details on their job requirements. Together, these factors can explain role conflict and ambiguity and the resulting stress among health care professionals working at the Fever Clinics [29]

The inverse association between social support and stress levels was expected. Two recent studies conducted on healthcare professional in Saudi Arabia showed that, during the COVID-19 pandemic, participants who did not perceive enough emotional support from society and the workplace had higher stress levels than those who perceived enough emotional support [29,37]. This finding elucidates the need to provide social support to healthcare professionals on the frontlines to improve their psychological health.

Of note, this study also showed that younger and non-Saudi healthcare professionals were more likely to report stress than their older and Saudi counterparts. The vulnerability of younger people to stress during the COVID-19 pandemic has been reported, highlighting the importance of tailoring mental health interventions for this age group [38]. The disparity in stress levels between Saudi and non-Saudi healthcare professionals can be attributed to the fact that non-Saudi healthcare professionals could not travel to their home countries because of the travel restrictions associated with the COVID-19 pandemic. It could also reflect a worse occupational environment or fewer financial motivations. However, this association should be further studied in future research.

5. Strengths and Limitations

This study had many strengths, including the multistage random sampling approach, using validated and reliable scales data to collect data on the work-related stressors and stress levels, and focusing on healthcare professionals in the frontlines managing COVID-19. Still, some limitations should be addressed. First, since the cross-sectional design cannot guarantee causality, studies with prospective designs are needed to confirm our results.

Second, the data collecting tool had no information on the lack of personal protective equipment, one of the significant stressors among healthcare professionals during the COVID-19 time. Third, we accessed participants using emails. Online surveys have many advantages such as cutting time, saving funds, decreasing missing data, yet they include some limitations such as the high possibility of non-response bias. Since we have no data on the nonrespondents, we cannot guarantee that the respondents had similar sociodemographic data and work-related stressors [39].

6. Conclusions

The current study showed that among healthcare professionals working at the Fever Clinics and managing COVID-19 in Saudi Arabia, role conflict and ambiguity were positively associated with stress levels. In contrast, social support was inversely associated with social support. We believe that the reasons behind role conflict and ambiguity among healthcare professionals in the Fever Clinics in Saudi Arabia should be studied, and tailored interventions should be put into practice.

Author Contributions: Conceptualization, S.A. and F.A.; data curation, S.A. and F.A.; formal analysis, S.A.; methodology, S.A. and F.A.; project administration, S.A.; supervision, S.A. and F.A.; validation, F.A.; investigation, S.A.; writing—original draft preparation, S.A., and F.A.; writing—review and editing, S.A., and F.A. All authors have read and agreed to the published version of the manuscript.

Funding: This research received no external funding.

Institutional Review Board Statement: The study was conducted according to the guidelines of the Declaration of Helsinki, and approved by the Institutional Review Board of Ministry of Health (protocol code: 31-30M and date of approval: 16 March 2021).

Informed Consent Statement: Not applicable.

Data Availability Statement: Data is available upon reasonable request by contacting the corresponding author.

Acknowledgments: The authors thank Khalid Al-Mansour for his permittance in using the data. Also, the authors also thank leaders of primary health centers and healthcare workers who participated and assigned a part of their time to this study.

Conflicts of Interest: The authors declare no conflict of interest.

References

1. World Health Organization. *Report of the WHO-China Joint Mission on Coronavirus Disease 2019 (COVID-19) Situation Report—93*; World Health Organization: Geneva, Switzerland, 2020; Available online: https://www.who.int/docs/default-source/coronaviruse/who-china-joint-mission-on-covid-19-final-report.pdf (accessed on 2 March 2021).
2. Zhou, P.; Yang, X.-L.; Wang, X.-G.; Hu, B.; Zhang, L.; Zhang, W.; Si, H.-R.; Zhu, Y.; Li, B.; Huang, C.-L.; et al. A pneumonia outbreak associated with a new coronavirus of probable bat origin. *Nature* **2020**, *579*, 270–273. [CrossRef]
3. World Health Organization (WHO). Mental Health and Psychosocial Considerations during the COVID-19 Outbreak—18 March 2020. Available online: https://apps.who.int/iris/rest/bitstreams/1272383/retrieve (accessed on 2 March 2021).
4. Adly, H.M.; Aljahdali, I.A.; Garout, M.A.; Khafagy, A.A.; Saati, A.A.; Saleh, S.A.K. Correlation of COVID-19 Pandemic with Healthcare System Response and Prevention Measures in Saudi Arabia. *Int. J. Environ. Res. Public Health* **2020**, *17*, 6666. [CrossRef] [PubMed]
5. World Health Organization. Corona Virus Dashboard: Saudi Arabia. 2021. Available online: https://covid19.who.int/region/emro/country/sa (accessed on 2 March 2021).
6. Al-Tawfiq, J.A.; Memish, Z.A. COVID-19 in the Eastern Mediterranean Region and Saudi Arabia: Prevention and therapeutic strategies. *Int. J. Antimicrob. Agents* **2020**, *55*, 105968. [CrossRef] [PubMed]
7. Al-Tawfiq, J.A.; Sattar, A.; Al-Khadra, H.; Al-Qahtani, S.; Al-Mulhim, M.; Al-Omoush, O.; Kheir, H.O. Incidence of COVID-19 among returning travelers in quarantine facilities: A longitudinal study and lessons learned. *Travel Med. Infect. Dis.* **2020**, *38*, 101901. [CrossRef]
8. AlJishi, J.M.; Alhajjaj, A.H.; Alkhabbaz, F.L.; AlAbduljabar, T.H.; Alsaif, A.; Alsaif, H.; Alomran, K.S.; Aljanobi, G.A.; Alghawi, Z.; Alsaif, M.; et al. Clinical characteristics of asymptomatic and symptomatic COVID-19 patients in the Eastern Province of Saudi Arabia. *J. Infect. Public Health* **2020**, *14*, 6–11. [CrossRef] [PubMed]

9. Saudi Ministry of Health. The Kingdom of Saudi Arabia's, Experiences: In Health Preparedness and Response to COVID-19 Pandemic. 2020. Available online: https://www.moh.gov.sa/en/Ministry/MediaCenter/Publications/Documents/COVID-19-NATIONAL.pdf (accessed on 2 March 2021).
10. Wang, C.; Pan, R.; Wan, X.; Tan, Y.; Xu, L.; Ho, C.S.; Ho, R.C. Immediate Psychological Responses and Associated Factors during the Initial Stage of the 2019 Coronavirus Disease (COVID-19) Epidemic among the General Population in China. *Int. J. Environ. Res. Public Health* **2020**, *17*, 1729. [CrossRef] [PubMed]
11. Roy, D.; Tripathy, S.; Kar, S.K.; Sharma, N.; Verma, S.K.; Kaushal, V. Study of knowledge, attitude, anxiety & perceived mental healthcare need in Indian population during COVID-19 pandemic. *Asian J. Psychiatry* **2020**, *51*, 102083. [CrossRef]
12. Xiong, J.; Lipsitz, O.; Nasri, F.; Lui, L.M.W.; Gill, H.; Phan, L.; Chen-Li, D.; Iacobucci, M.; Ho, R.; Majeed, A.; et al. Impact of COVID-19 pandemic on mental health in the general population: A systematic review. *J. Affect. Disord.* **2020**, *277*, 55–64. [CrossRef] [PubMed]
13. Galea, S.; Merchant, R.M.; Lurie, N. The Mental Health Consequences of COVID-19 and Physical Distancing: The need for prevention and early intervention. *JAMA Intern. Med.* **2020**, *180*, 817–818. [CrossRef] [PubMed]
14. Galbraith, N.; Boyda, D.; McFeeters, D.; Hassan, T. The mental health of doctors during the COVID-19 pandemic. *BJPsych Bull.* **2020**, *45*, 93–97. [CrossRef] [PubMed]
15. Alfawaz, H.; Yakout, S.; Wani, K.; Aljumah, G.; Ansari, M.; Khattak, M.; Hussain, S.; Al-Daghri, N. Dietary Intake and Mental Health among Saudi Adults during COVID-19 Lockdown. *Int. J. Environ. Res. Public Health* **2021**, *18*, 1653. [CrossRef] [PubMed]
16. Shigemura, J.; Ursano, R.J.; Morganstein, J.C.; Kurosawa, M.; Benedek, D.M. Public responses to the novel 2019 coronavirus (2019-nCoV) in Japan: Mental health consequences and target populations. *Psychiatry Clin. Neurosci.* **2020**, *74*, 281–282. [CrossRef] [PubMed]
17. Alsubaie, S.; Temsah, M.H.; Al-Eyadhy, A.A.; Gossady, I.; Hasan, G.M.; Al-Rabiaah, A.; Jamal, A.A.; Alhaboob, A.A.; Alsohime, F.; Somily, A.M. Middle East Respiratory Syndrome Coronavirus epidemic impact on healthcare workers' risk perceptions, work and personal lives. *J. Infect. Dev. Ctries.* **2019**, *13*, 920–926. [CrossRef] [PubMed]
18. Khalid, I.; Khalid, T.J.; Qabajah, M.R.; Barnard, A.G.; Qushmaq, I.A. Healthcare Workers Emotions, Perceived Stressors and Coping Strategies During a MERS-CoV Outbreak. *Clin. Med. Res.* **2016**, *14*, 7–14. [CrossRef] [PubMed]
19. Park, J.-S.; Lee, E.-H.; Park, N.-R.; Choi, Y.H. Mental Health of Nurses Working at a Government-designated Hospital During a MERS-CoV Outbreak: A Cross-sectional Study. *Arch. Psychiatr. Nurs.* **2018**, *32*, 2–6. [CrossRef] [PubMed]
20. Lazarus, R.S.; Folkman, S. Cognitive Theories of Stress and the Issue of Circularity. In *Dynamics of Stress*; Springer International Publishing: Boston, MA, USA, 1986; pp. 60–80.
21. Al-Omar, B. Sources of Work-Stress among Hospital-Staff at the Saudi MOH. *Econ. Adm.* **2003**, *17*, 3–16. [CrossRef]
22. Chekole, Y.A.; Minaye, S.Y.; Abate, S.M.; Mekuriaw, B. Perceived Stress and Its Associated Factors during COVID-19 among Healthcare Providers in Ethiopia: A Cross-Sectional Study. *Adv. Public Health* **2020**, *2020*, 5036861. [CrossRef]
23. Said, R.M.; El-Shafei, D.A. Occupational stress, job satisfaction, and intent to leave: Nurses working on front lines during COVID-19 pandemic in Zagazig City, Egypt. *Environ. Sci. Pollut. Res.* **2021**, *28*, 8791–8801. [CrossRef]
24. García-Herrero, S.; Lopez-Garcia, J.R.; Herrera, S.; Fontaneda, I.; Báscones, S.M.; Mariscal, M.A. The Influence of Recognition and Social Support on European Health Professionals' Occupational Stress: A Demands-Control-Social Support-Recognition Bayesian Network Model. *BioMed Res. Int.* **2017**, *2017*, 4673047. [CrossRef]
25. Maulik, P.K.; Eaton, W.W.; Bradshaw, C.P. The Effect of Social Networks and Social Support on Mental Health Services Use, Following a Life Event, among the Baltimore Epidemiologic Catchment Area Cohort. *J. Behav. Health Serv. Res.* **2011**, *38*, 29–50. [CrossRef] [PubMed]
26. Xiao, H.; Zhang, Y.; Kong, D.; Li, S.; Yang, N. The Effects of Social Support on Sleep Quality of Medical Staff Treating Patients with Coronavirus Disease 2019 (COVID-19) in January and February 2020 in China. *Med Sci. Monit.* **2020**, *26*, e923549. [CrossRef] [PubMed]
27. Thoits, P.A. Stress, Coping, and Social Support Processes: Where Are We? What Next? *J. Health Soc. Behav.* **1995**, *35*, 53. [CrossRef]
28. Norbeck, J.S.; Tilden, V.P. International nursing research in social support: Theoretical and methodological issues. *J. Adv. Nurs.* **1988**, *13*, 173–178. [CrossRef] [PubMed]
29. Al-Mansour, K.; Alfuzan, A.; Alsarheed, D.; Alenezi, M.; AboGazalah, F. Work-Related Challenges among Primary Health Centers Workers during COVID-19 in Saudi Arabia. *Int. J. Environ. Res. Public Health* **2021**, *18*, 1898. [CrossRef] [PubMed]
30. Faul, F.; Erdfelder, E.; Buchner, A.; Lang, A.G. Statistical power analyses using G* Power 3.1: Tests for correlation and regression analyses. *Behav. Res. Methods* **2009**, *41*, 1149–1160. [CrossRef] [PubMed]
31. Cohen, S. Perceived stress in a probability sample of the United States. The Claremont Symposium on Applied Social Psychology. In *The Social Psychology of Health*; Spacapan, S., Oskamp, S., Eds.; Sage Publications, Inc.: Newbury Park, CA, USA, 1988; pp. 31–67.
32. Bowling, N.A.; Khazon, S.; Alarcon, G.M.; Blackmore, C.E.; Bragg, C.B.; Hoepf, M.R.; Barelka, A.; Kennedy, K.; Wang, Q.; Li, H. Building better measures of role ambiguity and role conflict: The validation of new role stressor scales. *Work. Stress* **2017**, *31*, 1–23. [CrossRef]
33. Abu-Bader, S.H. *Using Statistical Methods in Social Science Research: A Complete SPSS Guide*, 2nd ed.; Lyceum Books, Inc.: Chicago, IL, USA, 2011.
34. Iverson, R.D.; Maguire, C. The relationship between job and life satisfaction: Evidence from a remote mining community. *Hum. Relat.* **2000**, *53*, 807–839. [CrossRef]

35. Zalaquett, C.P.; Wood, R.J. *Evaluating Stress: A Book of Resources*; The Scarecrow Press: London, UK, 1998; pp. 185–197.
36. Chiara, P.; Luca, C.; Annalisa, P.; Chiara, R.; Panari, C.; Caricati, L.; Pelosi, A.; Rossi, C. Emotional exhaustion among healthcare professionals: The effects of role ambiguity, work engagement and professional commitment. *Acta BioMed. Atenei Parm.* **2019**, *90*, 60–67.
37. Arafa, A.; Mohammed, Z.; Mahmoud, O.; Elshazley, M.; Ewis, A. Depressed, anxious, and stressed: What have healthcare workers on the frontlines in Egypt and Saudi Arabia experienced during the COVID-19 pandemic? *J. Affect. Disord.* **2021**, *278*, 365–371. [CrossRef]
38. Varma, P.; Junge, M.; Meaklim, H.; Jackson, M.L. Younger people are more vulnerable to stress, anxiety and depression during COVID-19 pandemic: A global cross-sectional survey. *Prog. Neuro-Psychopharmacol. Biol. Psychiatry* **2020**, *109*, 110236. [CrossRef]
39. Arafa, A.E.; Anzengruber, F.; Mostafa, A.M.; Navarini, A.A. Perspectives of online surveys in dermatology. *J. Eur. Acad. Dermatol. Venereol.* **2019**, *33*, 511–520. [CrossRef] [PubMed]

MDPI
St. Alban-Anlage 66
4052 Basel
Switzerland
Tel. +41 61 683 77 34
Fax +41 61 302 89 18
www.mdpi.com

Healthcare Editorial Office
E-mail: healthcare@mdpi.com
www.mdpi.com/journal/healthcare

www.ingramcontent.com/pod-product-compliance
Lightning Source LLC
LaVergne TN
LVHW070557100526
838202LV00012B/489